T0148584

ACUPOINTS

The Miracle Points Of Our Bodies

Dr Ravza Yausheva Veli

Translated by Ezel Jupiter

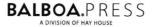

BALBOA.PRESS
A DIVISION OF HAY HOUSE

Balboa Press books may be ordered through booksellers or by contacting:

Balboa Press
A Division of Hay House
1663 Liberty Drive
Bloomington, IN 47403
www.balboapress.com.au
AU TFN: 1 800 844 925 (Toll Free inside Australia)
AU Local: 0283 107 086 (+61 2 8310 7086 from outside Australia)

Print information available on the last page.

ISBN: 978-1-5043-2339-0 (sc)
ISBN: 978-1-5043-2340-6 (e)

Balboa Press rev. date: 12/17/2020

Medical Disclaimer

This booklet is intended as an informational guide and is not meant to treat, diagnose, or prescribe. For any medical condition, physical symptoms or disease state, always consult with a qualified physician or appropriate health care professional. The author does not accept any responsibility for your health or how you choose to use the information contained in this booklet.

If you are currently under treatment with a qualified health practitioner, ask their advice before commencing any of the procedures in the book. If you are taking medication or other prescribed don't stop, unless on the advice of your health practitioner.

ACKNOWLEDGEMENTS

This book, which will take you on the journey of gaining your own health and helping your family's health step by step, was born with the touch of many people. I am so grateful for the many good people in this world. When you need help, they come with outstretched hands to assist you. For the following people, I want to offer my special thanks.

First to my kind-hearted and knowledgeable parents, I owe them gratitude for nurturing me through hardship and difficult times and providing for my education which has finally led to this book.

The next person who comes to mind is Prof. Dr. Fikret Turkmen (Izmir), my teacher and mentor, who gave me confidence and changed my life forever. He was also my Turkish language teacher.

Ms. Nurcan Akat (Istanbul) was the lead writer for Milliyet, the biggest newspaper in Turkey, and initiated the publication of the original publication of this book.

I also thank my wonderful friend Dilek Öngider, who guided me while writing, and raised me up every time.

There are three people who made this English edition of my book come true. I cannot thank them enough. All of them were nature's best gifts for me.

Ezel Jupiter (Sydney), she not only translated my book, she also helped me to persevere during some hard times. My love that gushed out from my deep heart, this love will always be with you!

Meredith Hamilton (Melbourne) was a great life coach for me. As well as the editor for the translation of my book for over a year. Discipline, patience, peaceful kindness, and sacrifice are in her soul. With her strong pen and style, my book will finally be presented to the world. Thank you so much!

I would like to express my many thanks to Andrew McLaren. The final edition of my book was developed and edited by him. He is a true professional who has made my book easier to read and understand with his knowledge of Chinese medicine and expertise as an editor.

Now I would like to express my special gratitude to two people. One is my dear son Ehset; He helped me with the images for this book but more importantly, he helped me understand the culture in this great country, Australia.

And my husband, Muslih. He is a wonderful friend and a faithful husband; He strives to be with me in every aspect of his life. He is one of the greatest blessings of this life for me.

PREFACE

Healthy living has become increasingly difficult for many of us. It is getting harder to find a natural lifestyle that we once had but seem to have lost. Away from nature, we experience stress-filled days and are constantly exposed to unhealthy living conditions. We are finding it difficult to find a patch of earth to walk on barefoot or to hug a tree when we are feeling down. In many places around the world, the balance of nature has been affected by the reduction in green space, climate change, radiation, air pollution, water shortages, drought, flood, and mass migration.

On the one hand, improved technology is providing us with endless possibilities, on the other hand it is removing our connection with nature and is causing health hazards to us as humans. We are challenged regularly and are often shocked when scientists prove that the habits, we believed were healthy are no longer recommended. For these reasons, more and more people are wanting to turn to nature for answers. They are rejecting western medicine, losing their faith, not finding cures for their illnesses and not recovering well after their illness.

We are well aware that there are alarming rates of disease, and generally unhealthy people all over the world. Are we taking it seriously though? Firstly for ourselves, then our families, our environment and even for our community. When we are not well, we jump around looking for safety like a chicken burning its feet on hot coals. This is a terrible situation. Wouldn't the health of the community improve if everyone learnt a bit about their own health, took care of it and managed to 'stop' or at least prevent illness before it happened? Wouldn't we live in a more peaceful environment?

In this book, I am not trying to tell the secret to a long life. I want to pass on my knowledge to people for health and quality of life for themselves, their families and their communities. I wish to find the lost balance in the world and to do something about it. From this book, what you will learn is that the energy 'streams' in your body can flow clearer and without barriers and this way, you will gain many good things that you may never have imagined. Some people may see it as an old-fashioned way, but this knowledge has been practised for thousands of years, contributing to our good health by natural methods. I say, let us use our bodies better to protect our health. What do you say to begin to look after yourself to maintain a healthy mind and body and build a healthier family and community?

According to Chinese Medicine, health means to be in a good condition physically, mentally and socially. Based on this definition, what percentage of our community is healthy do you think? When we look around, we see people complaining about tiredness, lack of concentration, lack of libido, forgetfulness, breathing problems, headaches, lack of appetite or eating disorders, fear and anxiety, anger, pain - the list goes on. People are not feeling healthy even if their issues are undiagnosed.

Many people find that western medicine is not helping them, so they ignore their symptoms, or worse, deny them. Now they are finding that, rather than taking a tablet or syrup, many symptoms can be relieved at home, for no cost, with no side effects. For example, after a long time seated at the computer, you can massage a point between the thumb and forefinger, called He Gu, to relieve blurred vision and stiff neck.

Similarly, massaging a point on the inside of the arm just up from the crease of the wrist, called Nei Guan, can relieve nausea.

You will find in this book details of the points I use in my practice and teach my clients to use at home, the symptoms they relieve, and the techniques for achieving maximum benefit. Remember these points are not treatments for disease. They give temporary relief in most cases. For more serious concerns, or if symptoms persist, you must speak to your qualified health practitioner.

How this book came about

I grew up in a different culture and where I lived, in Urumqi China, people used different methods to protect their health. I learnt Traditional Chinese Medicine as well as traditional Turkish methods, having arrived in Turkey when I was 35 years old. I was fortunate enough to take part in a television program there where I gave the audience clear, practical and helpful information. Viewers began contacting me, asking me: "Where can we buy your book?"

So, I started writing in Turkish. The work was tiring but it gave me happiness, love and enjoyment. I was sharing my 38 years of knowledge and experience with the wider community. The book was published in Turkey in 2009. Since then, it has been republished 5 times.

My husband and I have lived in Australia for three years now, where I have continued my health practice in The Block Arcade in Melbourne. I am very happy to have this book revised and translated into English to reach a wider audience.

In this book you will find theories for a healthy life, acupressure points for everyday use, breathing exercises, massages that you can do yourself, and advice based on Traditional Chinese Medicine. There is something for everyone. If you take it seriously and practice regularly, miraculous things can happen. You can discover that those tiny points can produce unbelievably big results. Believe in them and work on them. You will then find happiness, health, comfort, self-confidence and success. I recommend it to all people who care about their health. I feel so pleased to share this with you. I love everyone. I love all of humanity. I love the earth with all its contents. And I know that people who know love will be loved. Love yourself.

You and your body are always wonderful!

Dr Ravza Veli

CONTENTS

Chapter 5   Signs, Symptoms and Solutions 97

INTRODUCTION

In the 21st century health and wellbeing is paramount in people's minds. We are opting for a broader view of what we need to do to stay healthy and how we treat ailments when they arise.

There is no single medical regime that can treat or cure everything. That is why many doctors of western medicine are incorporating complementary disciplines in their practice or working together with other practitioners to achieve the best outcome for their patients.

As alternatives to western or orthodox medicine, many people are turning to natural or complementary healing modalities such as naturopathy, chiropractic, Ayurveda and reiki. One of the most effective of the alternative disciplines is Traditional Chinese Medicine (TCM), nowadays referred to simply as Chinese Medicine.

The first chapter of this book is devoted to explaining Chinese Medicine and its place in the health care system.

Acupressure uses the same points as acupuncture. Whereas in acupuncture we use needles, for acupressure we use our fingers to massage. The points used in these methods of treatment are a foundation of Traditional Chinese Medicine.

Why are the acupoints important?

The acupoints and meridians are based on strong theory, and philosophy developed over many centuries. For thousands of years, this philosophy has become stronger and proved itself. It continues to prove itself through good results. The theory behind the acupoints and meridians accepts the body as one and does not deal with ailments such as headache, loss of hair or back pain as separate problems. It does not examine one area but looks at the whole body when diagnosing an illness. With this method, not only is the area of complaint treated but also other future complaints are prevented. This is done by keeping the Yin and Yang balanced at an optimum level which heals and makes the person feel strong and healthy.

Using the acupoints and meridians of the body can assist in maintaining good health and people can see the results in their lives. It is easy to practice, is low cost and has hardly any side effects. When using the acupoints, if people pay attention to the points and the method of application, it will work sufficiently to care for the wellbeing of the whole body. Once learned, patients can recognise or diagnose symptoms and solve some of their own issues. It does not have a negative impact on ongoing treatment. In fact, in some cases where western medicine is unsuccessful, working with the acupoints may actually effect a cure. It provides support to current treatments and is often referred to as complementary medicine. It can be used at any stage of life. Most importantly, doctors and patients in the West now see the benefits of the points and meridians. People began to study the points and now everyday more and more people are using meridians and acupoints to maintain their health and wellbeing.

What is Chinese medicine?

Chinese Medicine is more than an effective medical treatment. It is a philosophy. The foundation of Chinese Medicine - concepts of Yin and Yang, the Five Elements Theory, Qi, and meridians - are difficult to prove. They are seen by many practitioners as a metaphor to explain how and why Chinese Medicine works.

It does work. Thousands of peer-reviewed papers by authors around the world, published in respected scientific journals attest to its efficacy. Most aspects of the success of Chinese Medical treatments are explained by current physiological knowledge.

In recent years many people around the globe have been placing more importance on their health. They are aware of what is happening around them. The increase in cancer, heart disease and diabetes, among other diseases, causes concern. People do not want it to happen to them. They struggle to find a way to maintain a healthy lifestyle. The healing techniques of Chinese Medicine have been used for many thousands of years and help us to have a better quality of life. Knowledge of the meridians and acupoints does not cost any money, does not have any side effects, does not require any external assistance, and it can help improve our wellbeing.

Acupuncture and acupressure, the application of needles or massage to particular, well-defined points on the body, area major aspects of Chinese medical treatment. This book describes some of the techniques that practitioners use that anyone can do for themselves at home.

You will get from this book a comprehensive understanding of the philosophy and techniques of TCM, with an emphasis on the acupoints. Many descriptions, symptoms, treatments and procedures are explained in TCM terms. When we talk about heat, water stagnation, flow of Qi, meridians, and the like, they are translations of Chinese words and phrases and should be read in this context. There is a glossary at the end of the book to explain them.

Qi is a name for the vital energy that flows throughout our bodies through well-defined meridians or channels. Although they cannot be seen directly, they have been shown to exist.

Sometimes the meridians become blocked or the flow of Qi is sluggish, causing various symptoms. The acupoints are locations on the meridians that allow us to regulate the Qi, helping to restore the balance of Yin and Yang.

Two chapters are devoted to describing the locations and functions of some important acupoints, and the symptoms that they will relieve. I would like to point out again that this book is an educational guide. **For persistent or serious symptoms, you must see a qualified practitioner**, whether it be western medicine, Chinese, or another discipline of your choice.

In my years of practice, I have developed a system that fully incorporates the application of acupressure with other established health modalities. It is called Ra Qi. There is an entire chapter about it. I am very proud of it and have achieved some major successes. Ra Qi is unique to my practice.

The body of this work ends with my philosophy and suggestions for a healthy life – physically, mentally, spiritually and emotionally.

The Duty and Obligations of a Medical Practitioner

You have no doubt heard of the Hippocratic Oath. Hippocrates was a doctor in Greece around 2500 years ago. He was the first to recognise that disease came from internal and external factors, and not by visitations from the gods.

The premise of his oath is 'First do no harm'. The welfare of the patient is paramount.

The Australian medical profession swears a similar oath. Although I am not, nor claim to be, a registered medical practitioner, the sentiment resonates with me so well I feel moved to reprint it here.

I solemnly pledge to consecrate my life to the service of humanity; I will give to my teachers the respect and gratitude that is their due; I will practise my profession with conscience and dignity; The health of my patient will be my first consideration; I will respect the secrets that are confided in me, even after the patient has died; I will maintain, by all the means in my power, the honour and the noble traditions of the medical profession; My colleagues will be my sisters and brothers; I will not permit considerations of age, disease or disability, creed, ethnic origin, gender, nationality, political affiliation, race, sexual orientation, social standing or any other factor to intervene between my duty and my patient; I will maintain the utmost respect for human life; I will not use my medical knowledge to violate human rights and civil liberties, even under threat; I make these promises solemnly, freely and upon my honour.

(Declaration of Geneva, WMA, 2006)

CHAPTER 1
Chinese Medicine

Traditional Chinese Medicine (TCM) is practised and influenced by Chinese traditional culture. It is built on the foundation of many thousands of years of study and practice. It applies both the Chinese medical science and Chinese herbal medicine to protect human life functions as well as to diagnose illnesses and provide treatment.

Traditional Chinese Medicine sees the human body as one and applies the concept of Yin and Yang, and the Five Phases theory. It investigates the causes of ill health, characteristics and its location by looking, smelling, questioning and checking the pulse. The investigation looks for changes in the organs, meridians, energy flow, blood and body fluids. The diagnosis is based on what illness is present and what is lacking.

By the application of these treatments, the body's positive balance is achieved, and health is recovered. Chinese Medicine gives as much importance to spiritual health as it does to physical health. Chinese Medicine practitioners still refer to the ancient medical text by the Yellow Emperor Nei Jing which is also used to help people become moral and respectable.

The foundation of Chinese Medicine is the re-balancing of Yin and Yang. We must maintain this balance so as not to allow the decline of our health, and to have a strong organism - a healthy human body. There are five fundamental modalities of treatment. They are:

- Diet
- Acupuncture and Moxibustion
- Herbal medicine
- Exercise
- Massage

They are so integrated that each one incorporated facets of the others. They all work to the same end. Restoring balance of Yin and Yang, and regulating Qi to achieve harmony within the body to restore and maintain good health.

Chinese Medicine attends to the patient rather than the disease. Diagnoses are made on the basis of determining the causes and nature of imbalances.

Yin and Yang

The classic Chinese ideology of Yin and Yang is where philosophy and medical science meet. It is known as profound science. It explores the connections and the contrasts between all creation. For example; male and female, happiness and unhappiness, full and hungry, darkness and light, hot and cold, night and day, up or down, moving or stationary, black or white, sick or healthy.

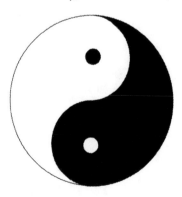

There are five meanings to this symbol.

1. For all things in nature, there exists an inseparable and contradictory opposite to each other. They are characterised by Yin and Yang. These opposite and contrary forces must complement and interconnect with each other in order to continue their existence in the natural world. For example, heat belongs to the Yang group, and cold to the Yin group. These two factors exist in continuous battle with each other. As applied to our bodies, the upper part is Yang, the lower part is Yin. Our outer skin is Yang, inner is Yin, hollow organs are Yang, filled organs are Yin, Liquids are Yin, air and gas are Yang. Every organ has Yin and Yang elements. In Chinese medicine, the theory of Yin and Yang is used in clinical work and diagnosing the human organism, its functions and pathological changes.

2. Their existence of each depends on the existence of the other. In Asian philosophy, "Yin will not exist without Yang, Yang will not function without Yin". This proverb is well known. We said the upper part is Yang, the lower is Yin. Because there is an upper, we can make a reference to it to describe the lower. To talk about hot, we feel its opposite cold. In our organism the substance is known as Yin, and the function is Yang due to its activity. The function exists as it is the indicator of the substance.

3. They exist in using each other. The human body is a being formed by a relative balance of Yin and Yang (by providing an active balance). If our body balance is out of order, our organs cannot function in an orderly manner and either we get sick or our quality of life drops. The physiological function of the organism will work and maintain its relative balance with Yin and Yang harmony. Fluids (blood and various other body fluids) are necessary to feed our organs to function normally. Again, for the nourishing fluids to

exist, the organs need to work. In this way, our organism in continuous connectivity is in action to help us maintain a balanced living. We must remember one thing here: Our bodies are always trying to keep their balance depending on our environment, our nutrition and our spiritual changes we experience. Therefore, we need to apply constant protective action. We need to listen to our bodies' small signals and we must act to protect our health.

4. Yin and Yang can completely change. What was Yin can turn into Yang, or Yang can turn into Yin. This is an unbalanced and diseased change. We can illustrate this with an example: To have a fever is a Yang illness (body temperature is rising). If the organism does not find a cure, it will keep rising. It can reach a point in which the body potentially cannot bear it and will start dropping. Yin and Yang will lose their balance and the pulse will drop, the skin will lose colour, hands, and feet will become cold and the blood pressure will drop. These are the signals for Yin illness. In this situation, if the correct treatment is used, the person will get out of the Yin and will move towards Yang. The pulse will improve, the colour will return to the face, hands and feet will warm up and the patient will begin recovery. The fevered body becomes cold. This is an example of the body turning Yang to Yin. If it changes from Yin to Yang the results are indicating improvement.

5. Inside a Yin there is always Yang, and inside Yang there is always Yin. They will be in existence this way infinitely. To understand the human organism, Chinese Medicine studies the body in two Yin and Yang groups. As explained above, the Yin and Yang theory is used in understanding how the organs work, to notice the pathological changes, in diagnosis and to see how the illness is progressing. It assists in deciding the treatment and it may change in line with the progress.

ACUPOINTS

The Organs

There are two important differences in the way Chinese Medicine refers to organs compared to the way most westerners regard them.

The first is that Chinese Medicine practitioners consider the anatomy and the function as a whole, inseparable from each other. Furthermore, the function of the organ is considered to be far more than the physiological function as viewed by western medicine.

The second is that Chinese Medicine sees two entities as organs that are not regarded as such in western medicine. One is the pericardium, a protective envelope of tissue around the heart. The other doesn't exist in physical form at all. It is called the San Jiao (Triple Burner). It is described fuller in Chapter 2.

The Meridians

In the last twenty or more years, many people around the world have become interested in the Body Meridians. We can say that the meridian is a multi-level, multi-functional, multi-dimensional three-dimensional structure control system. In Traditional Chinese Medicine, the meridians are very important because knowing about them is like having the owner's manual for the human body.

We have 14 main meridians in our bodies. Two of which are single and central. The other twelve are bilateral, duplicated on each side of the body. Each one links to a certain organ and body part. Energy (Qi) currents exist inside the meridians, so they are referred to as energy channels. Each meridian carries the energy to the area or the organs it is linked to. If we have any illness or a problem with any of our organs, sensitivity or pain can occur at the points of the corresponding energy channel. This would signal that an issue is developing. We must pay attention to and take care of these organs. A well-known Chinese proverb says, "If there is a blockage, there will be pain and sickness". Caring for the channels is similar to working the soil with a hoe, giving us the oxygen we need.

Chapter 3 describes the meridians, their connections with each other and between the parts of our bodies.

Qi

TCM considers three factors that comprise the human being. Called the Three Treasures, they are Jing (the Essence), Qi (energy), and Shen (the Soul). This book concerns itself with Qi.

The principle of Qi is the basis of all energy in Traditional Chinese Medicine. It is much more than what English speakers understand by energy, however.

When we look at the way Qi is written in classic and modern Chinese. As we know the Chinese script is made up of characters and as such, each character may have more than one meaning.

炁 contains both 无 (absent/does not exist) and 火 (fire) that the absence of fire or the anger fire, means there is Qi. It is not hard to understand that when there is no anger there is a lot of energy. In addition, the word 'energy' takes on 氣 to mean air, gas, wind, strength, move, power and further with 气 meanings such as rice, food, feed, and takes shape with the giver of life 米.

From this word, we can understand that if we are breathing, we will take in oxygen and have a balanced diet, we will always have energy. In fact, we use and feel this shapeless, colourless, odourless thing called energy that is impossible to touch, everywhere, every day. For example; heat, electricity, fire, flame, movement, breath and the excitement we feel are all energy.

There are different types of Qi, with different qualities. I will explain some of them here as they pertain to Chinese Medicine in general, and acupoints in particular.

The Movement of Qi

The four directions of Qi movement are up, down, outward, and inward. These movements are so important that once Qi can no longer travel in these directions, life will end.

Each organ has different specialised movements. For example, spleen Qi ascends the pure part of digested food from the stomach for transformation into nutritional essence. Stomach Qi, on the other hand, pushes food downwards in order to remove its impurities. Some organs, like the lungs, perform movements in all four directions. Lung Qi moves in and out during breathing.

The different movements of Qi work in a coordinated manner to maintain a harmonious balance. The ascending balances the descending movement while the outward balances the inward movement. Balanced movement is important for promoting the physiological functions of different tissues, organs, and meridians. The disharmonious movement of Qi leads to health problems. For example, an insufficient downward movement of lung Qi causes a cough. When stomach Qi cannot descend, nausea, and vomiting occurs.

Types of Qi

Original (inborn, Vital) Energy (Yuan Qi)

We can also call this the root energy and the life force; it is the most important energy in human life. It is the energy we bring with us as we are born from our mother's womb. This main energy source is stored in our kidneys. It feeds our internal organs to function and makes us dynamic. After birth, its continuous power is supported by water, food, breathing, sun, nature and various other energy sources.

Pectoral Energy (Zong Qi)

Zong Qi is provided from nature by breathing. It is believed to come from cosmic sourced energy. Also named as the big energy, it creates a pushing force in the breathing function. Zong Qi affects speech, tone of voice, strength of our breath, and sense of smell. Its push force affects the heartbeat and rhythm and body temperature. Oxygen is its base; it can be strengthened by breathing correctly and through breathing exercises. Pectoral energy is stored in our lung

Nutritive energy (Ying Qi)

This energy supplies nourishment to the body. It comes from food and becomes stronger through good nourishment. It mainly circulates through the blood vessels with the blood. Nutritive Qi has yin properties so it can form into materials needed by other parts of the body. For example, its close relationship with blood allows it to provide some of the necessary substances needed to produce new blood. Ying Qi controls organ functions. It helps with the brain, hand and foot movements. Ying Qi moves all the nutrition to the organs, but the organs can only take the matter at the time allocated, and not when they need it. We can think of this as a metabolic process. With the right food choices, we can make this energy stronger.

Defensive Energy (Wei Qi)

The meaning of the word *Wei* is to protect. It relates to protection and defence of the body. It takes its power from grains. Wei Qi moves outward from the body to repel invasive pathogens. Strength of the bones, hair and skin indicates that the Wei energy is strong. If the Yang energy is sufficient then the Wei energy will be strong, and the pores will be open. In this case the energy exchange is easier, and the energy is used more effectively. If the Yin energy is more than the normal level, the Wei energy will fall, and the pores will close. In this case, the body's defence will become weaker, the hair will look weak and will fall out. The skin will look dull. This energy protects us from cold and heat.

The Four Seas

TCM considers that there are four seas that comprise various acupoints are associated with four systems in the body.

1. Energy Sea - centred in the chest, affects the amount and flow of Qi
2. Grain Sea - in the upper abdomen, is the main area for energy production
3. Blood Sea - in the area called Dan Tian (about 2-4 finger widths below the navel), it is the body's centre of energy)
4. Marrow Sea - inside the skull, the essence of our energy reserve.

The seas are not unlike the chakras of Hindu philosophy.

In summary, without Qi there is no life. There is only to add here that the strength and vitality of Qi is also affected by emotions. For example, sadness diminishes Qi. We protect and invigorate our Qi by maintaining proper nourishment, keeping warm when it is cold and cool when it is hot, and controlling our emotions.

Acupuncture, Acupressure, the Acupoints, and Moxibustion

Along each meridian there are specific locations that are susceptible to manipulation by a skilled practitioner. Just as valves and inspection ports are located at strategic points along a pipeline.

According to Chinese Medicine, stimulation with needles, massage or moxa (see below for a description of moxibustion) at these points can

> ➤ clear a blockage that is inhibiting the Qi from flowing, or
> ➤ stimulate the flow of sluggish Qi
> ➤ augment or build up Qi

These are the acupoints. They are small energy centres on the meridians that contain special healing and treatment powers and can protect us from illness. The practice of using these points for diagnosis and treatment is called *Zhen Jiu*.

Moxibustion is the practice of using a dried plant called Moxa (mugwort) used to heat the needle for use in acupuncture or to activate the points directly. Cupping therapy, healing stones and magnets are also used on some points. With the advancement in technology, laser and electronic acupuncture is often use. These do not involve skin penetration and eliminate the risk of infection. Some practitioners believe that they are not as effective.

The main effects of the acupuncture points are:

1. They are used in examination for diagnosis as the points can reflect the illness

2. They are used to treat illnesses
3. They impact on the energy as they are the energy entry and exit points, so they can improve our energy
4. They can protect the body from illness and improve immunity

About Acupuncture

Acupuncture involves the use of needles to activate the acupoints. The most common method is the use of silver, steel and gold needles. As modern practice is to use needles only once, steel needles are most commonly used.

Traditional Chinese Medicine believes that acupuncture leads to restoring Yin and Yang balance, stimulates the points, dispels toxins (poisonous matter) from the body, clearing energy blockages, opening meridians, increasing the body's defence system, or balancing the immune system. Whatever the theories are, we know that the body can repair its own systems.

In acupuncture training, we know that acupuncture has benign and bi-directional stimulation effects on the same acupoint. For example, if you apply acupuncture to people who sweat too much, the sweat will be reduced. If you treat people who complain that I don't sweat at all, then if you treat them with the same acupoints, the body will start to sweat. The same point can warm up the area that is cold, or cool down the area that is too hot, and the same acupoint can reduce or increase the amount of menstruation.

As the worldwide use of acupuncture is increasing there is more understanding of the effects of the points. There has been much scientific investigation into why acupuncture has been successful so often. Some theories that have been postulated are

> An increase in endorphins and enkephalin that help reduce pain in the body following an acupuncture treatment.
> An increased natural healing hormone or neurotransmitter secretion in some cases of allergy or depression. The patient's belief that this healing method will help them and a placebo effect occurs.
> The body's electric flow may change after the application of these methods.

Research shows that acupuncture treatment and point stimulation can result in health recovery in humans without side effects. In Chapter 4 we will learn about 60 points that you can use to treat various symptoms. I will explain those which are easily found and most commonly used.

Moxibustion

Moxa is a Chinese Medicine herb that is commonly known as mugwort. The herb is dried and then burned to produce a mild heat. Using moxa is a means of augmenting Qi. It is used in two ways. Practitioners of acupuncture attach a small plug of it to the end of a needle after it has been inserted at an appropriate acupoint. They then light the moxa, which smoulders with a gentle heat to increase the stimulation brought about by the needle.

The second use, more appropriate to this book, is to use either a stick of compressed moxa, or fill a specially made device and apply the heat directly to the point.

The Five Elements

The Five Elements are inseparable factors of Yin and Yang. They are talked about in unison in the Chinese philosophy - Yin and Yang and Five Elements.

These theories, with the pure materialist ideas of classical Chinese, were the way of recognising nature as they came. They tried to understand the nature within the Yin and Yang theory by grouping the matters into the tree (wood), water, fire, metal, and earth (soil). They researched their relationship to one another, their formation and effects. As a result, the strong theory and the work principles that used around the world today came to exist.

The phrase Five Elements is a means of classifying the nature of various entities - be they material objects, people, emotions, natural or observed phenomena - into one of five groups. Each group has a specific nature. Certain inferences can be drawn by knowing the Five Element nature of say a person.

The Five Element Theory does not imply that everything in the universe is made of the five elements. In times gone by there was a belief (in Europe, not in China) that everything in the universe was made by a combination of some or all of fire, water, earth and air. Some English-speaking practitioners prefer the term Five Phases.

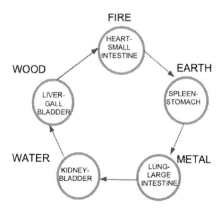

The Five Elements and the Relationship with Our Organs

Within the framework of the Five Element theory There is a complex interplay between the organs. Each organ generates Qi for the following in cycle. On one hand the organs support each other, and on the other hand they control and regulate each other. Thus, is shown how all the organs are interrelated. TCM believed this fitted in with the law of nature as human beings are part of nature. For thousands of years the human body was researched in this way by TCM masters. They learnt, for example, which organs need 'water' or not, which organs need to be rid of 'humidity', or which are prone to 'fire'. This way helped them decide how to protect and treat their patients. These methods of prevention and treatment generally change with the improvements in treatment.

The treating doctor will change and apply treatments or preventions to the patient by following and checking the natural changes occurring along the way. Thus, a practitioner may determine a problem in the kidney may be due to a deficiency in the lung, which is the generating organ. So, they will build up the lung before treating the kidney problem. Only by keeping an eye on the reactions of the body can correct treatment and protection techniques be applied. Let's now meet the five elements in our bodies.

The following table shows the five elements and some of their associated attributes.

ELEMENT	WOOD	FIRE	EARTH	METAL	WATER
COLOUR	GREEN	RED	YELLOW	WHITE	BLUE
SOLID ORGANS	LIVER	HEART	SPLEEN	LUNG	KIDNEY
HOLLOW ORGANS	GALL BLADDER	SMALL INTESTINE	STOMACH	LARGE INTESTINE	URINARY BLADDER
TISSUES	TENDON	BLOOD VESSEL	MUSCLE	SKIN and HAIR	BONE
SENSES	EYE	TONGUE	MOUTH	NOSE	EAR
EMOTIONS	ANGER	JOY	OVER THINKING	GRIEF	FEAR
PRINCIPLES	TRUST	RIGHTEOUSNESS	PROPRIETY	WISDOM	COURTESY
TASTES	SOUR	BITTER	SWEET	SPICY	SALTY
DIRECTION	EAST	SOUTH	CENTRAL	WEST	NORTH
SEASONS	SPRING	SUMMER	LATE SUMMER	AUTUMN	WINTER

CHAPTER 2
The Organs

The Organs according to Chinese Medicine

Chinese medicine groups the organs into five *Zang* (solid), six *Fu* (empty) and *Qi Heng Zhi Fu* groups.

The five Zang organs are; lungs, liver, heart, spleen, and kidneys.

The empty organs are: stomach, large intestine, small intestine, bladder, and San Jiao (Triple Burner).

In addition, a group called *Qi Heng Zhi Fu* (extraordinary) includes brain, marrow, bones, blood vessels and reproductive organs. Due to their function, they are grouped separately.

These 11 organs plus the Pericardium, which is a protective tissue surrounding the heart, constitute the 12 meridians described in Chapter 2.

In Chinese Medicine there is an entity called San Jiao, translated as Triple Burner or Triple Warmer. This is not an organ at all in western medical terms. It is not part of the anatomy. Nevertheless, it performs vital functions in Chinese Medicine and thus has a meridian dedicated to it. It comprises three parts - upper, middle, and lower - as described below.

As mentioned in the introduction, when Chinese Medicine talks about an organ it includes the function of that organ, in Chinese

Medical terms, as well as the anatomical organ. Form and function are inextricably interconnected.

Lungs: Manage the energy, breathing, ensuring the blood vessels are open to protect the heart. Control the pores. It opens in the nose and links to the large intestine, connects to the skin and its fluid is the mucus. Its feeling is longing.

Heart: Controls the function of blood and vessels. Controls emotions. It belongs to the fire group. It is connected to the small intestines. It begins in the tongue. Its fluid is sweat, and its colour reflects on the face. Its sense is love.

Pericardium: Protects the heart. Classical Chinese thought there was a container that protects the heart outside of it. This "cap" is not only protecting the heart but also with its own meridian it ensures the energy flows without a blockage. It affects human psychology with its connections to three heating meridians.

Spleen: It is known as the main source of strength. Together with the digestive system, it converts water and food into goodness for life function. It cleanses the blood and provides blood to other organs in its best, most useful form. It controls the blood quality. It is placed within the earth group and connects to the stomach and muscles. It opens in the mouth, its fluid is saliva, its colour is reflected in the lips.

Liver: Its main function is to distribute the blood and store it. It ensures the body functions without congestion. It impacts on the nutrients to be absorbed by the body. Its feeling is anger. If it is well looked after it ensures a good mood. The liver is the organ that is affected most by anger. It belongs to the wood group and connects to the gallbladder. It opens in the eye, its fluid is the tear, links to tendons, its colour reflects in the nails and the eyes.

Kidney: The kidneys' main function is to hide the jewel for body energy, growth and reproduction functions. The kidney is the centre of Yin and Yang, core storer and the source of life. The Kidney produces marrow to provide life support to the body, and links to the bladder. It belongs to the water group; its colour reflects in the hair. If the hair is strong and shiny the kidneys are full of energy. Its feeling is fear.

Gallbladder: The gallbladder links to the liver and belongs to the wood group. Gall liquid(bile) is produced and stored in it. This liquid enters the small intestine and helps digestion. It affects decision making. Its colour reflects in the eyes.

Stomach: The stomach belongs to the earth group which links to the spleen. They are together the foundation of strong health and wellbeing. Its function is to receive the food and cook it, supplying energy and passing it downwards. It supports the whole energy channels to remain open with its push power.

The spleen and stomach together provide the material basis of the acquired constitution.

Small intestines: The small intestines belong to the fire group and link to our heart. Its main function is to receive the food from the stomach and digest it. It will store needed nutrients and will discharge the rest.

Large intestines: The large intestines belong to the metal group and link to the lungs. The function to receive the discharge from the small intestine and will make it harden by removing the liquid. It will then pass the liquid to the bladder.

Bladder: The bladder belongs to the water group and links to the kidneys. Its function is to store urine and discharge it.

San Jiao: This organ is very hard to understand by western people. It does not belong to the five elements. In Chinese medicine, this organ is known as the carrier of energy flow, consisting of three parts:

Upper Jiao: The top part of the diaphragm, aids to increase and distribute the energy.

Middle Jiao: The empty space between the diaphragm and the abdomen. Together with the organs in this area, it forms the axis and it is the source of energy and blood production. The stomach, spleen, liver and gallbladder are located in this space.

Lower Jiao: The Small intestines, large intestines, kidney, and bladder are located in this space. It is believed that the essence of life is kept here. Nutrients that are necessary are saved and waste is sorted to be discharged. It is known as the safe cup of the organs.

Brain: Its physiological functions include consciousness, mind, thinking, intelligence, sight, smell, hearing, and taste, as well as speech, and movement. The brain is the extension of marrow. The marrow makes the brain strong. The marrow is the 'ore' produced by the kidney. If the function of the kidney is weak, the marrow nucleus will not be balanced, and the marrow will not be made. Lack of marrow will unbalance the brain function and weaken it. This can result in slowed reaction times, the retreat of intelligence, slurred speech, a feeling of emptiness and tiredness. To keep the brain in balance, firstly the kidneys, then the other organs need to be well looked after.

Marrow and bone: The marrow is inside the bone and its main function is to produce blood, feed the bone for its development and feed the brain to keep the whole body in balance. The marrow's formation depends on kidney function. If the kidney is not producing enough nutritive essence, the marrow will remain weak. This will lead to health complaints of the brain and body.

The light reflecting on the face will show the marrow's strength. The skeletal system gives shape to the human body and keeps it upright against gravity. To have strong bones, strong kidneys are needed. The strength of our bones can be observed from people's walking style (gait), posture and other functions like movement.

Blood vessels: The blood vessels are the channels and 'the palace' for blood and its movement. The channels should be open for healthy blood flow and energy. Many illnesses can present when the blood thickens, or its content is not healthy, the energy is weak or the veins are damaged. Chinese Medicine pays a lot of attention to the notion that "If there is a blockage, there is illness".

Blood Vessels contain blood. Blood is produced from marrow which is produced from kidney essence and also from the transformation of food Qi with the help of the original Qi of the kidney. Thus, the blood vessels are indirectly related to the Kidneys.

We can understand this with the vascular system in western medicine. There are three major types of blood vessels: arteries, capillaries, and veins. Capillaries consist only of a layer of endothelium and occasional connective tissue. This structure allows the exchange of water, nutrients, and chemicals between the blood and the tissues. Arteries carry oxygenated blood away from the heart. They are composed of three layers of tissue. Most veins carry deoxygenated blood from the tissues back to the heart with the exception of the pulmonary and umbilical veins, both of which carry oxygenated blood to the heart. The location of veins is much more variable from person to person than that of arteries. Many veins are located close to the skin, whereas arteries run deeper.

Uterus: Its main functions are to regulate periods and carry out pregnancy. To carry out these, all other organs need to be working in order. Most importantly, the kidneys must function well and the abdomen energy must be well stored.

Each organ is associated with a meridian, either directly or indirectly. The following chapter fully describes the meridians, and their link with the organs.

CHAPTER 3
The Meridians

The meridians are channels that carry Qi. There are 12 meridians that pertain to the organs. They form a closed loop, as each has a connection with the meridian before and after it. Each one has an interior and a surface component, with branches to connect with other meridians and organs. They are symmetrically bilateral. The surface branch exposes the meridian to treatment at certain points, the acupoints.

There are also two vital meridians that form a loop along the longitudinal midline of the head, chest, back and abdomen. They are the Ren Mai (Conception Vessel) and Du Mai (Governing Vessel).

The 12 Meridians

Lung Meridian

Flow line:

1. Starts internally at the centre of the abdomen, passes through the stomach, diaphragm and lungs.
2. Passing through the lungs and trachea it comes to the surface, passing below the collarbone, through the shoulder, down the inside arm, finishing 2 mm behind the thumbnail.
3. It branches at the fork between thumb and forefinger to meet the large intestine meridian.

Function: This channel carries Yin energy. It is used in the treatment of lung and skin and other illnesses affecting the organs and tissues in its passage. It is also important and used to increase the body's defences by protecting it from respiratory diseases and skin problems.

Illness signals: The signals of imbalance in the Lung Meridian generally occur in the throat, chest and respiratory tract. Fullness in the chest, shortness of breath, pain in the upper part of the collarbone, pain in the arm and back, chill (not liking cold), burning of the palm, feeling tired (due to lack of energy), skin problems and allergic reactions are common findings.

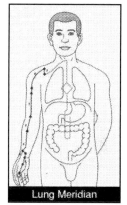

Lung Meridian

Large Intestine Meridian

Flow line:

1. Starts at the medial (thumb facing) side of the forefinger, then passes through the wrist, traveling upwards through the elbow, reaching the shoulder.
2. One of its branches passes through the diaphragm and links to the large intestine
3. After passing through the neck the other branch reaches the face linking to the mouth and teeth, finishing between the nose and the edge of the lip, where it connects with the Stomach meridian.

Connected organs: Lungs and Stomach

Function: This meridian keeps the large intestine's balance and works to ensure that body waste is discharged effectively and timely. It also keeps the electrolytes in balance.

Illness signals: Generally, when the large intestine meridian's balance is disturbed the complaints are around the head, face, ear, nose, mouth and tooth. It shows extreme heat. The most common complaints are, toothache, rhinitis, common cold, dryness of the mouth, throat ache, face itching, pain, redness and watering of the eyes, neck and shoulder pain, pain in the arms, feeling warm and bloated, fever and shivering, feeling pain and hardness in the fingers.

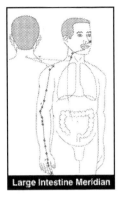

Large Intestine Meridian

Stomach Meridian

Flow line:

1. Starts at the edge of the nose and reaches to its top-end where it meets the eye and joins with the bladder meridian.
2. It travels downwards from both sides of the nose, then reaches the chin, circles the lips, to the chin again
3. Here it branches past the front to the hairline, and descends down the neck, through the chest and abdomen (diaphragm and stomach).
4. It then passes through the groin and down the outside of the leg, through the knee, alongside the tibia (shin), through the front of the ankle, along the top of the foot, finishing at the outside of the second toe.

Connected organs: Spleen, heart and small intestine

Functions: It keeps the stomach balanced to accept and keep secretions, maintain digestion, as well as carrying and emptying functions. It provides energy to the body. It positively affects the body's wei qi and immune system. It also impacts on the heart and the small intestine's work either positively or negatively as it is linked to both meridians.

Illness signals: Generally, when the stomach meridian's balance is disturbed, the complaints are around the head, nose, teeth, throat, brain and digestive systems. Stomach pain and bloating, an increase in appetite, throat infection, nasal flow, cold and flu, yawning too much, anxiety or being easily affected by sounds, tachycardia, face paralysis, mouth and tongue sores, apoplexy, increased body heat are common complaints and sicknesses.

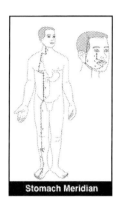

Stomach Meridian

Spleen Meridian

Flow line:

1. Starts at the back of the big toenail, moving upwards from the inside of the ankle bone it passes through the inside of the tibia to the groin.
2. It passes to the abdomen and connects with the stomach, travels upwards passing through the diaphragm, continues up the throat and ends under the tongue.
3. Another branch coming out of the stomach passes to the diaphragm, flows to the heart and makes a connection.

Connected organs: Spleen, heart and small intestine

Functions: The stomach and the spleen are connected organs. The Spleen Meridian's energetically balanced work ensures that digestion is working in balance. The Spleen Meridian provides heat balance to organs supporting their functions. It provides the nutritional materials to the body. It is also effective in ensuring blood quality.

Illness signals: Any imbalance in the Spleen meridian shows up in the stomach and intestines. Feeling of swollen and hard tongue, loss of appetite, indigestion, losing weight, stomach pain, bloating, constipation or diarrhoea, not getting taste from food, too much burping, passing gas, feeling body weight, dull skin, swelling and pain of the knee, and anaemia are amongst the major complaints.

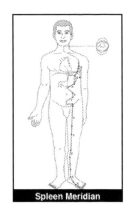

Spleen Meridian

Heart Meridian

Flow line:

1. Starts from the armpit, passes through inside and middle of the arm downwards, across the palm, ending at the little finger.
2. A branch passes through the throat and reaches the eye.
3. Another branch enters the abdominal cavity.

Connected organs: Small intestine, lungs, spleen, liver and kidneys

Functions: It reacts to signals it feels. It controls the entire body as the "Sea of Energy". It can motivate people by producing energy or consumes energy and pulls people down. When it flows well, it gives us the feeling of peace, affection, confidence.

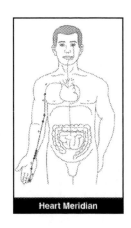

Heart Meridian

Illness signals: Imbalance of the Heart Meridian generally affects the person's mental health. Unhappiness, lack of sleep, loss of confidence, strain, indecision, dry mouth, palpitations, heavy chest, sweating at night, pain inside of the arm, sweaty and burning palms are common findings.

Small Intestine Meridian

Flow line:

1. It starts from behind the fingernail of the little finger, along the medial side of the hand and ulna and the back of the arm to the back of the shoulder.
2. It then crosses the scapula, up the side of the neck and across the face to the cheek bone, finishing in front of the ear.
3. It connects with the bladder meridian at the edge of the eye.

Connected organs: Heart and stomach

Functions: This is a blood-rich but energy-poor meridian. It keeps the small intestine's balance for its absorption and secretion work. It supports our body for the food to turn into nutrition. It is also known as the "Heart function mirror" due to the connection between the intestine and the heart. Care of this meridian is very important as it supports the small intestine and the heart.

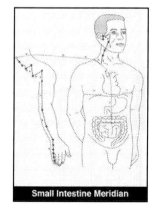
Small Intestine Meridian

Illness signals: Imbalances of the small intestine usually present in both sides of the head, cheeks, arm, ear and may affect mental health. Sore throat, swollen cheek or jaw, ringing in the ears, hard of hearing, pain in the area of the arm where this meridian is passing, difficulty in movement and feeling of hardness, pain or numbness in the pinkie, and hot flashes are some of the common complaints.

Bladder Meridian

Flow line:

1. It starts at the inner canthus of the eye, moves up the forehead to the hairline, continuing along the top of the scalp, down the back of the head, where it branches down the neck.
2. The two branches run parallel adjacent to the spine, through the buttock, down the back of the leg, where they meet behind the knee. In the abdominal cavity it connects with the kidneys.
3. It then runs down the back of the lower leg, around the lateral malleolus (outside ankle), along the side of the foot, to finish at the little toe where it meets the kidney meridian.

Connected organs: Kidney, heart and brain

Functions: The bladder meridian is our body's largest channel of waste materials. It is similar to our cities' sewage systems and continuously carries waste. From head to toe, it collects the waste and sends it to the bladder to be expelled. Due to its connection with the Kidney meridian, its work is connected to the work of the kidney. We need to look after this channel if we do not want the toxins to accumulate in our bodies.

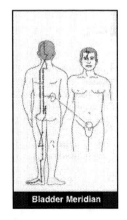

Bladder Meridian

Illness signals: Bladder meridian imbalance will mostly show in the eye, nose, head and neck, back and waist and brain. Headache, stiffness of the neck, waist and back pain, problems with the eyes, nose drip, pain in the hipbone, cramping of the little toe, coldness or hotness in the legs, irregular menstruation, complaints relating to stress are the common complaints.

Kidney Meridian

Flow line:

1. Starts at the little toe. The first acupoint is on the sole of the foot.
2. It then comes around the inside of the foot, circles the medial malleolus (inside ankle), rising up the inside of the leg.
3. It ascends the front abdomen and thorax to the collar bone, connecting with the vertebrae, the bladder, the kidney and the diaphragm.
4. Another branch reaches the lung and the heart.
5. It passes through the throat and ends under the tongue.

Connected organs: Bladder, liver, lung, heart, bone, hair and body hair

Functions: The Kidney Meridian is the main channel that brings health and happiness. The quality of life can be high if this meridian is healthy and strong. According to the Chinese medicine "the kidney is the main genetic organ and a life investment". The kidney meridian positively works in the production of our body energy, purification of waste, increasing our body's resistance to disease. Shiny hair and skin and strong bones are the indications that the kidney meridian is open.

Illness signals: The imbalance of the kidney meridian will generally show in the reproductive system, lower abdomen and intestines. Sometimes it occurs with throat and lung complaints. Losing appetite a lot, dull skin, losing the shine in the eyes, being out of breath following a low level activity, head spin, unwillingness, being tired all the time and wanting to sleep, anxiety, dry and hot mouth and throat problems, the coldness of hands and feet and not being able to warm up are the common complaints due to poor circulation.

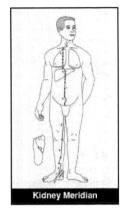

Kidney Meridian

Pericardium Meridian

Flow line:

1. Begins inside the chest. Passes through the pericardium connecting with the top, middle and lower warmer (San Jiao) in the abdomen.
2. A branch from the chest reaches the armpit circles around the armpit, goes downwards through the inside of the arm.
3. It goes downwards from the centre of the front of the arm.
4. Passing through and reaches the palm, ending at the end of the middle finger.
5. A branch in the palm of the hand at the ring finger makes the connection with the Triple Burner meridian.

Connected organs: The three meridian's passage areas and the pericardium.

Functions: It is known for its connection to a person's mental health. It is important that this meridian is continuously flowing for a person to be happy and peaceful. It is very important for heart health.

Illness signals: Hot and sweaty hands, elbow pain, pain under arm, restlessness, physiological imbalance, extreme red face, chest pain and feeling of fullness, depression, palpitations, sleep problems and hot flashes.

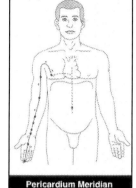

Pericardium Meridian

Triple Burner Meridian

Flow line:

1. Begins at the edge of the ring fingernail, along the top of the fourth and fifth finger across the back of the hand through the wrist.
2. It passes between the ulna and radius, along the inside of the humerus, reaching the shoulder, where it branches.
3. One branch travels internally, passing through the pericardium and diaphragm uniting the Triple Burner.
4. The other branch passes up the side of the neck, rises from behind the ear, circles the ear, finishing at the outer end of the eyebrow where it connects with the Gall Bladder meridian.

Connected organs: Pericardium and all the organs in the abdomen area

Functions: In Chinese Medicine, there is an additional organ that is known as the 'San Jiao'. It is like a big bowl that fits all the other organs inside. We can see this as our body torso. It divides this into three Jiao. We can say it is three parts of the torso. The upper Jiao contains the heart and lungs, the middle Jiao contains the stomach, spleen, and gallbladder. The lower Jiao contains the kidneys, bladder, small and large intestines.

According to the theory, we call this the Triple Burner (Three Jiao) Meridian providing energy and coordinating functions to all the organs. We can see the Triple Burner meridian as the conductor of the orchestra and the organs are the musicians. If the conductor does a good job the orchestra produces good music. In other words, for the organs to work in harmony is made possible by the triple burner energy providing them with good energy evenly. Its work is also recognised for keeping the body temperature in balance and carrying the nutrition across the body. It is hard to understand this meridian as it is not seen by the eye. In the past, people used to see it as "an open window' for their benefit. You can see an amazing view from an open window if you want to. But sometimes we try to see the window using other people's eyes, other perspectives and we say: "Show it to me, what's there?" Maybe we can see more things if we use our eyes and also try to see from another's perspective.

The only thing we need to know here is a meridian on the outer surface of our arm; If we take good care of it, if this meridian works well, our organs will work well. We can see much healthier organs through our "Three Jiao windows".

Illness signals: A loss of balance of the Triple Burner meridian generally shows around the head, throat, chest. Ringing in the ears or loss of hearing, infection in the throat, headache, cheek and chin pain, pain on the outside of the eye, shoulder pain, sweating at night, pain on the outside of the elbow, restlessness, restricted movement of the ring finger are common concerns.

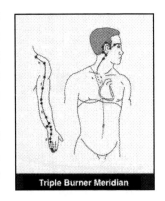

Triple Burner Meridian

Gallbladder Meridian

Flow line:

1. Starts at the outside corner of the eye, flows to the front and back of the ear, traverses one side of the scalp three times front-to-rear, then down the neck to the shoulder
2. From the collarbone cavity it passes down the flank, continues down the side of the abdomen, connecting to the diaphragm, the liver, and the gallbladder.
3. It then circles the genitalia, crosses to the rear of the hip, then down the side of the leg, passing in front of the lateral malleolus, finishing at the little toe.
4. A branch splits to meet the Liver Meridian.

Connected organs: Liver and heart

Functions: it has a positive impact on gallbladder fluid production. Specifically helps for lipid metabolism to be in balance. If we don't want to be overweight, we need to pay special care to this meridian.

Illness signals: An imbalance of the gall bladder meridian generally shows around the head, eye, ear, nose, chest and the sides of the body. Migraine, bitterness in the mouth, gall bladder illness, digestion problems, pain in the hips and back, sciatica, knee pain, infection of the milk glands, inability to produce milk after birth, period problems are common concerns.

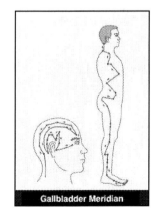

Gallbladder Meridian

Liver Meridian

Flow line:

1. Starts at the top of the big toe, flows along the top of the foot to the ankle.
2. It passes in front of the medial malleolus, up the inside of the leg, passing through the reproductive organs to reach the lower abdomen
3. Connects with the liver, the gallbladder, and the diaphragm.
4. In the abdomen it connects with the Lung Meridian, thus completing the full cycle of the meridians. On the surface it rises up the side of the abdomen and chest, the side of the throat and face.
5. It passes the inner canthus of the eye, up the forehead, to the vortex (top point) of the head.
6. A branch from the cheek curves around the inner surface of the lips.

Connected organs: Lungs, stomach, kidney, brain and it has a connection to the gallbladder.

Functions: The liver is the body's detoxification factory. The function of the liver is to store the blood and regulate the body's blood. When a person is moving, the liver will exhaust the blood of nutrients to support the body's needs. While resting and sleeping the need for blood is less and the liver deposits into the blood. For this reason, quality sleep is very important for the liver.

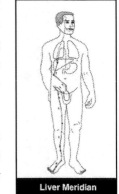

Liver Meridian

Illness signals: A blockage in the liver can cause our body's 'spring' energy, meaning the life energy to drop or disappear. Anger or unwillingness, cold or hot feet and hands, tiredness, dull skin, sexual problems, bloating, eyesight problems, period pains, chest pain, headache, shortage of breath and digestive complaints happen.

Ren Mai and Du Mai

Ren Meridian

'Ren' means 'direction, responsibility'. The Ren Meridian, the 'Conception Vessel', has a major role in Qi circulation, monitoring and directing all the Yin channels. It is the channel that takes all the Yin energy in the body and assumes the distribution task.

Flow line:

It starts in the abdomen and near the anus from the 'Hui Yin' point surfaces. It flows upwards from the genitals. It reaches the throat from the centre of the torso. It ends at the bottom of the lips. Its branch winds around the mouth and splits into two, connecting to the eye.

Functions: It is the main source of energy production and its storage. It ensures that the person is energetic and strong. It is crucial for keeping the Yin and Yang balance and distribution of the heat.

Illness signals: An imbalance of the Ren Meridian can impact the body's yin energy. Incontinence, impotence, unwillingness, disharmony, period problems, heavy flow, reproductive problems, bloating and pain, cyst, stomach pain, speech problems and numbness are common complaints. Blockage of its energy can cause a psychological withdrawal.

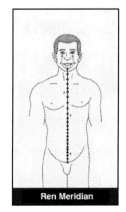

Ren Meridian

35

Du Meridian

Also called the Governing Vessel, the Du Mai is the 'Sea of Yang'. The Du Mai directs, nourishes, and monitors all the Yang meridians.

Flow line: Starts below the coccyx, then upwards along the surface of the spine, along the midline of the scalp, centrally down the face to finish inside the upper lip.

Functions: It connects directly with the brain and the spinal cord. The Du meridian energy flows through the spine, so it is our pole (pillar). Therefore, it is very important that we must protect our spine and the Du meridian. We will be healthy and strong if our Du meridian is strong.

Illness signals: Illness signals: Our yang energy is negatively impacted when the Du meridian is imbalanced. Common complaints include lower back pain, premature ejaculation, ejaculation while sleeping/dreaming, heavy menstruation, lack of libido, shortness of breath, feeling hardness in the spine, and headaches. Blockage of the energy results in an excessive reaction.

Summary

The Du and Ren are the single trunk meridians. They run up the front and back of the body line. They are easy to use and give excellent results. These two meridians resemble the trunk of a tree. They feed the leaves of the tree, keeping its balance.

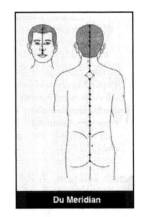

Du Meridian

The Meridian Clock

While Qi is continuously flowing through the meridians, it is stronger in each meridian at certain times of the day.

Every organ in our bodies carries out the work without us noticing while we are living our daily lives. We do not need to think about vital living functions like digestion, absorption, breaking down of toxins and expelling from our bodies, or the creation of energy. Our organs work like a clock, based on their role continually doing their work. However, we can negatively affect this regular system by imperfect work and life practices. Unbalanced living and daily disorder break down the working order of our organs and affects their functions negatively. Thus, the overworked organ may begin to break down and we get sick.

If we followed the clock of our organs, if we gave it importance, we would be healthier. In recent years, a 'Time Therapy' was developed that considered this matter. To do this effectively, we need to learn about our organ's working clocks and respect them to live better and healthier.

The following describes the times when Qi is strongest in each organ. Convention starts with the Lung Meridian.

03:00 – 05:00, The Lung meridian

At this time, the lungs are working at their highest potential. The lungs clean and expel matter mostly during this lung time. People who cough will cough more between these hours. The window should be slightly open between these hours. When I was a child there was a small window over the large one that would be kept open through the night. Nowadays we need to open the large windows. To help the meridian of the lung, we find a way to get fresh air.

DR RAVZA YAUSHEVA VELI

05:00 – 07:00, Large intestine meridian

We should empty the large intestine around this time. If we don't do this, the toxic matters accumulate in our body and can make us ill later. It may even cause weight gain. Once we miss the morning toilet, we lose the feeling of going to the toilet during the day and may result in constipation.

The large intestine depends on the lungs for movement via the expansion and contraction of the diaphragm, which works like a pump to give impetus to peristalsis by regulating abdominal pressure.

07:00 – 09:00, Stomach meridian

This is the stomach working hour. We must have breakfast to provide our body with the energy it needs for the day. Don't skip breakfast.

09:00 – 11:00, Spleen meridian

11a.m is the spleen hour. In Chinese Medicine, the function of the spleen organ-energy system includes the pancreas. Called the 'Minister of the Granary'. The spleen and pancreas control extraction and assimilation of nutrients from food and fluids by providing the digestive enzymes and energy required by the stomach and small intestine. We must have breakfast in time if we want the spleen to work well.

11:00 – 13:00, Heart meridian

This is the most delicate hour for the heart. It is called the 'King' of the organs because the heart controls our emotions. Controlling our emotions is important in these hours.

13:00 – 15:00, Small intestine meridian

This is the peak hour for the small intestine doing its work. The small intestine receives partially digested food from the stomach and further refines it, separating the pure from the impure', then assimilating the purified nutrients and moving the impure wastes onwards to the large intestine for elimination. Its energy meridian runs into the head, where it influences the function of the pituitary gland, the 'master gland' whose secretions regulate growth, metabolism, immunity, sexuality, and the entire endocrine system. Drinking a glass of water will support it. Anger must be avoided.

15:00 – 17:00, Bladder meridian

We should not hold on to urine at this time. The bladder meridian is the longest meridian in our body. As an energy system, the bladder Meridian is intimately related to the functions and balance of the autonomic nervous system.

17:00 – 19:00, Kidney meridian: This is the peak hour for the kidneys to do their work. Chinese medicine knows the kidney as the 'Root of Life'. It is the most important organ in terms of energy production. TCM sees the kidney is an organ system which also includes the adrenal glands, the testicles in men and the ovaries in women. During these hours, it is important to keep the waist area warm; not hold on to going to the toilet, and to avoid extreme tiredness.

19:00 – 21:00, The Pericardium meridian

This area is known as the time of the day when blood pressure is highest and fluctuates easily. We should avoid activities that would negatively affect our feelings. This is a pleasant time to spend with family or friends. This would be very beneficial to the pericardium.

21.00 – 23.00: San Jiao meridian (Triple Burner)

Not a single self-contained organ, but rather a functional energy system involved in regulating the activities of other organs. This is the best time for the immune system to work. It is important to rest. Breathing exercises, listening to music, reading and meditation would be very beneficial at this time.

23:00 – 01:00 Gallbladder meridian

The gallbladder governs daring and decisiveness. If we want this organ to work well, we must guarantee the quality of sleep. Even if possible, deep sleep at this time will come even better. It would be very beneficial for this body system not to drink and smoke.

01:00 – 03:00, The Liver meridian hour

Liver will work best when we are in a deep sleep. To go to sleep early and wake up early would protect the liver and be very beneficial. If you get up during these hours, you need to drink a cup of water, which will support the liver.

CHAPTER 4

The Location and Benefits of Acupoints

In this section, I talk from my experience gained from more than 30 years of work as a TCM practitioner. You can be sure that every acupoint you learn from here will bring you healing benefits. You may also find that the knowledge you gain will benefit not only yourself, but also your loved ones and the people around you. With the magic of the knowledge of the miracle points of your body, you'll be able to help others and create a healthier family and community around you. What a wonderful purpose to bring into your life!

When you are learning the points, remember that they appear twice on our body (on both sides), the only single points are the back and front midline points. Are you ready? Let's begin!

Here are some instructions on techniques to use with the acupoints.

How to Massage the Acupoints

1. *Finger pressure*

   Use your fingers, and the pressure is appropriate to the strength you can accept. Avoid too hard pressure.

2. Joint pushing

Make a fist and push with the joints of your fingers. It is suitable for harder parts, such as the lower limbs.

3. Empty fist beating lightly

Touch the tips of thumb and forefinger together and curl the fingers, as though holding a rod. Beat the point lightly with the circle made by the thumb and forefinger.

4. Friction massage

Use the palm surface, or index finger, middle, ring, and little finger, to do clockwise or counterclockwise circular movement gently rubbing.

5. Point method

Use your fingers to press on the acupuncture points. Take care to protect your fingers and avoid excessive stretching or bending.

Benefits of Massage

➢ It speeds up the blood circulation. It dilutes the blood and reduces stickiness.
➢ Lowers peripheral vascular pressure, so the burden of the heart decreased.
➢ The tempo and depth of breath change positively, more oxygen is supplied to the organs.
➢ Movement in the stomach and intestine increases. Improve digestion, absorption, and excretion.
➢ Emptying of the bladder becomes easier.
➢ Massaging acupoints can adjust hormone secretion balance.

> ➤ Calms the brain and body.
> ➤ Reduces stickiness, spasm, and oedema in the muscles.
> ➤ Revitalises the skin.
> ➤ Meridians are opened, the flow of energy becomes easier, raising the level of Qi.
> ➤ It reduces pain by reducing oedema around joints.

How to use moxa

Hold a burning moxa stick close to, but not touching, the surface of the skin.

In this method, the moxa material is compressed into a stick or pole, looking not unlike an oversized cigar that can be lit and allowed to smoulder, producing a unique form of very penetrating heat.

The smouldering moxa stick is held over specific areas, often, though not always, corresponding to certain acupuncture points. The glowing end is held about an inch or two above the surface of the skin until the area reddens and becomes suffused with warmth.

The Cun - measurement for locating acupoints

The system of using the *cun* is a way to measure and locate acupoints on anyone's body. Since everyone's body is of a different size and shape, using a person's inborn measurement system makes finding the points a snap.

The process starts with the measurement of one cun. This is done two ways:

1. using the width of the distal interphalangeal joint of the thumb (first finger), or
2. using the distance between the distal and proximal interphalangeal joints of the 3rd (middle) finger.

All other specific measurements are outlined in the diagrams below. When in doubt, you can use the thumb (1 cun) or the four-finger method (3 cun).

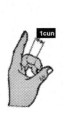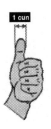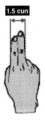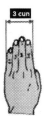

Acupoints: Location and Techniques

Points of the Lung Meridian

LU-5, Chi Ze (尺泽)

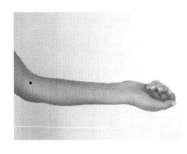

Location: At the cubital crease on the radial side of the biceps brachii tendon.

How to find the pressure point: Sit down and open your palm with the palm up on the table, raise your palm up a bit. Here you will find a pit on the thumb side of the tendon of your elbow you are feeling. This the pit which is the point we seek.

Benefits: Pressing this point is effective in preventing respiratory tract disease and ensuring complete lung function. Expels phlegm from the lungs. Prevents getting cold. Nourishes kidneys and skin.

Indications: Bronchitis. Cough. Fullness in the chest. Difficulty breathing. Swollen limbs. Enuresis (urinary incontinence). Relaxes the sinews in this channel path.

Method of Application: Start breathing deeply, when breathing out, rub or press the points with the thumb.

Breathing deeply again, continue the same process for 12-18 times. If available, Moxa is applied for 10 – 15 minutes.

Note: If you drink a cup of warm water before and after the massage, it will help to remove toxins.

LU 7, Lie Que (列缺)

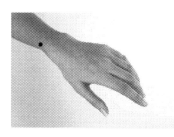

Location: 1.5 cun above the wrist crease.

How to find the pressure point: The left hand is lifted with thumbs up, and the palms are held towards yourself. The right angle of the thumb is placed at the same angle as the left hand. The point of the index finger is the desired point.

Benefits: Because of the meridian to which it is connected, it helps prevent or reduce symptoms of the common cold, cough, headache and shortness of breath. It is especially effective in smoking cessation.

This point is extremely useful in the complaints that are left after fractures and injuries due to the artery underneath. Opens the nose. Clears sadness. Repression of feelings.

Indications: Headache and stiffness of the neck. Cough and asthma. Sore throat. Facial paralysis. Dryness of the eyes and mouth Clenched jaws. Weakness of the wrist.

Method of Application: 12-18 times with the index finger massage the points. If available, Moxa is applied.

LU 10, Yu Ji (鱼际)

Location: On the thenar eminence, midway along the first metacarpal.

How to find the pressure point: Along the first bone of the thumb, between the muscle of the thumb and the bone.

Benefits: It helps prevent or reduce symptoms of the common cold, cough, sore throat, headache and shortness of breath.

Indications: This point helps the capillary in the region improves blood circulation. It has a direct positive effect on the vocal cords. It is good for hoarseness and loss of voice (also called aphonia).

Method of Application: 12-18 times with the index finger massage the points. If available, Moxa is applied.

LU 11, Shao Shang (少商)

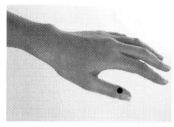

Location: 0.1 cun anterior to the 1ˢᵗ thumbnail radial corner.

How to find the pressure point: In the upper part of the thumb, 2 mm near the nail.

Benefits: Affects the direct breath, helps the breath to work in balance. Allows more oxygen to go to the lung.

Indications: Shortness of breath. Fever. Cough. Sore throat. Tonsillitis. Has a special effect on hiccups.

Target area: Throat.

Method of Application: Press the points with the thumb tip 12-18 times. The massage can be a bit difficult. It can be applied by putting Vaccaria seed (王不留行籽) or wheat grain on the point to create more feeling.

Points of the Large Intestine Meridian

LI 4, He Gu (合谷)

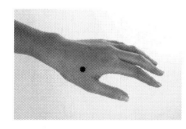

Location: In the middle of the 2ⁿᵈ metacarpal bone on the radial side.

How to find the pressure point: The point is located at the highest point of the muscle when thumb and index fingers are held together.

Benefit: When we talk about acupuncture, one of the first points that comes to mind is the He Gu point. The massage for this point creates a detox effect, increasing the amount of blood to the brain. It provides pain relief and has a calming effect. It keeps the bowel function in balance. It affects the neck and head positively. It is a kind of analgesia and is an important point where good results can be obtained to heal many diseases.

Indications: Analgesic. Anxiety. Headache. Fever. Regulates transpiration. Spasms in the stomach and intestines. Toothache. Blurred vision after a long time on the computer. Stiff neck. Cold. Flu. Rhinitis. Style. Facial paralysis. It gives the brain clarity. Good for colds.

Method of Application: Pressing 12-18 times massage of the points. Moxa is applicable for 10-15 minutes.

Note: Drinking a cup of warm water before and after the massage, will be more beneficial for removing toxins.

LI 11, Qu Qi (曲池)

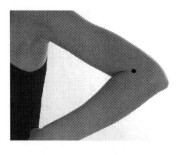

Location: At the lateral end of the transverse cubital crease midway between LU5 and the lateral epicondyle of the humerus.

How to find the pressure point: Curl the elbow, the end of the line formed in the elbow is the point we are looking for.

Benefit: Nourishes the skin, detoxifies. It is effective in smoking cessation. Clears Heat. Cools the blood (if yang energy is excessive)

Indications: Internal heat (Feel overly hot). Anger. Fever. Itching. Arm pain. Matting and fading skin. Skin diseases. Sunstroke. Constipation. A regular warming to this point ensures that the skin is always alive. Very useful for Menopause hot flushes.

Method of Application:

With the thumb tip 12-18 times pressing the points. The massage can be a bit stiff. Moxa is applicable for 10-15 minutes.

Note: Drinking a cup of warm water before and after the massage will be beneficial to remove toxins.

Points of the Stomach meridian

ST 2, Si Bai (四白)

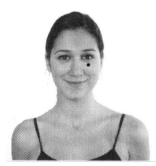

Location: Just below ST1, on the depression of infraorbital foramen.

How to find the pressure point: On the face, the point is directly below the pupil of the eye, in the depression at the infraorbital foramen.

Benefit: Enlightens the eyes. Clears the eye. It is useful for protecting eye function.

Indications: Some eye problems. Eyestrain. Night blindness. Blurred vision. Redness and swelling in the eye. Reduce Under-eye bag formation.

Method of Application: Tapping with the ring finger for 1-3 minutes. Can be tapped at the same time on both sides.

Note: Hands must be very clean, the tapping should not be too hard.

ST 4, Di Cang (地仓)

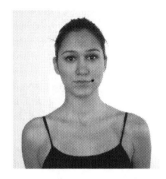

Location: At the meeting point of the vertical line passing through the centre of the pupil and the horizontal line through the corner of the mouth.

How to find the pressure point: 2 mm to the corners of the lip.

Benefit: Helps to secrete saliva. It stimulates the distribution of nutrients from the stomach, it provides hot energy to the body. Helps stabilise the stomach function. It is highly effective to balance the digestive system. Eating more slowly can have a positive effect on the appetite of anorexic people. Gives a feeling of satiety, helps lose weight. It is also useful in delaying the lines formed around the edge of the lips.

Indications: Trigeminal neuralgia. Swelling and numbness of the lips and face. Facial paralysis. Pain in the cheeks and teeth.

Method of Application:

Sit down, have a glass of warm water half an hour before a meal. Keep the lip slightly open. Fix the elbow on the table. Tapping the points for 12-18 times.

This massage should be done slowly.

ST 25, Tian Shu (天枢)

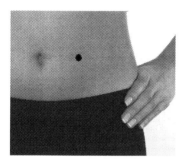

Location: 2 cun lateral to the umbilicus.

How to find the pressure point: In the middle of the abdomen, the three fingers to the right and left sides of the belly.

Benefit: It has a key effect on the intestines. It increases the resistance against disease and ensures the regular operation of the large intestine. Increases the body's ability to fight against colds. Regulates the intestines, stomach and Spleen. Eliminates humidity. Clears the Mind.

Indications: Digestive gas. Distention and abdominal pain. Constipation. Chronic diarrhoea. Swelling on the face. Irregular menstruation, menstrual cramps.

Method of Application:

Lying on your back. Massage on this point with four fingers. Take a deep breath, the fingers are free while breathing, and apply pressure while exhaling. Apply this process to each side 6 to 12 times. We can work it with two hands at the same time.

If available, Moxa is applied for 10 – 15 minutes.

Note: A glass of warm water before massage, will be beneficial.

Attention: Pregnant women and menstrual period should not use this point.

ST 36, Zu San Li (足三里)

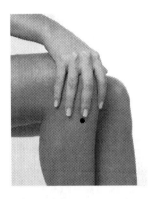

Location: 3 cun below the lower border of the patella, one finger width lateral from the anterior border of the tibia.

How to find the pressure point: Open your palm, the fingers pointing down, place the palm on the middle of the kneecap, the middle finger touches the point where it touches.

Benefits: This is one of the most researched acupoints. It is one of the most important protective points. It strengthens the energy of the stomach and spleen. It distributes the food as nutrients to all parts of the body in a balanced way. It is also effective in protecting against cardiovascular diseases.

Indications: Epigastric pain. Digestive difficulties. Fatigue. Dizziness. Blurred vision. Abdominal distension and pain. Feeling fullness and distention in the abdomen.

Method of Application: Tapping or pressing the points 12-18 times. The touch can be a little strong, as this is a hard area. Moxa is applied for 10–15 minutes.

Points of the Spleen Meridian

SP 1, Yin Bai (隐白)

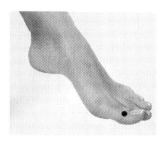

Location: On the medial side of the big toe 0.1 cun posterior to the corner of the nail.

How to find the pressure point: It is located on the inside of the two toes, 2 mm from the big toe.

Benefits: Balances the energy circulation in the spleen meridian. Control the quality of blood structure. Provides the removal of negative energy that needs to be removed from the body. It is effective in sending nutrients to organs. Regulates the Spleen. Stops bleeding. Calms the Mind.

Indications: Abdominal distension. Diarrhoea. Vomiting. Unwillingness to eat. Mental agitation and depression. Sigh. Sadness. Manic-depressive disorder. Excessive dreaming. Insomnia.

Method of Application: With the thumb tip 12-18 times pressing the points. The massage can be a bit stiff. If available, Moxa is applied for 10 – 15 minutes.

SP 6, San Yin Jiao (三阴交)

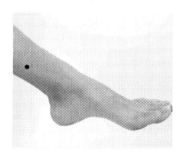

Meaning: Three Yin Meeting

Location: 3 cun directly above the tip of the medial malleolus on the posterior border of the tibia.

How to find the pressure point: Inside the lower leg, four fingers up on the ankle, on the inner side of the tibia, between the bone and the shin.

Benefits: I use this point on most of my patients. It is a very special point because the spleen, liver and kidney meridians intersect here. Because of this, the single point, balances the function of the three meridians. Strengthens the Spleen. Resolve the body's dampness. Stimulates the function of the liver. Smooths the flow of Liver Qi. Tonifies Kidney. Nourishes the Blood and Yin. Benefits urination. Regulates uterus and menstruation. Cools the blood. Stops pain. Analgesia. Calms the Mind.

Indications: Deficient Spleen and Stomach. Heaviness. Oedema. abdominal fullness and distension or bloating. Feeling cold in the abdomen. Navel pain. Dizziness. Irregular menstruation. Difficulty urinating. Enuresis (incontinence). Pain in the penis. Insomnia. Shyness. Irritability. Regular vaginal secretion. Night sweating. The sensation of heat.

Method of Application: With the thumb tip pressing the points for 3-5 minutes. The massage can be a bit stiff. If available, Moxa is applied for 10-15 minutes.

SP 8, Di Ji (地机)

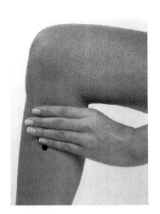

Location: 3 cun directly below SP9.

How to find the pressure point: On the inner part of the lower leg, above the ankle, 4 fingers below the Yin Ling Quan (SP9) point.

Benefits: Boosts immunity. Distributes nutrients from the spleen. It is a point that balances the energy flow of the spleen meridians, blood structure and supports the immune system. Ensures that the food we receive is acceptable to the body. Ensures the transformation of food into nutrients. Helps increase and dissipate the energy. Keeps the quality of blood in balance, gives colour to the lips. Enhances sense of taste. Nourishes and strengthens muscles.

Indications: Abdominal distension (bloating). Abdominal pain. Poor appetite. Irregular menstruation. Painful and excessive menstruation. Oedema.

Meridian: Spleen

Method of Application: With the thumb tip pressing the points for 3-5 minutes. The massage can be a bit stiff. If available, Moxa is applied for 10-15 minutes.

SP 9, Yin Ling Quan (阴陵泉)

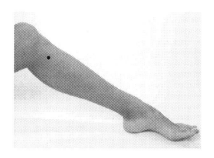

Location: On the lower border of the medial condyle of the tibia in the depression posterior and inferior to the medial condyle of the tibia.

How to find the pressure point: The index finger pushes up the inside of the calf, a cavity under the knee joint is the point.

Benefits: Collects and strengthens the energy in the spleen meridian. It helps the spleen to work properly. Distributes excess moisture, dissipates excess fluid in the body.

Indications: Abdominal distension and pain. Poor appetite. Diarrhea. Edema. Swelling in the legs. Enuresis (incontinence). Feeling fatigued.

Method of Application: With the thumb tip pressing the points for 3-5 minutes. The massage can be a bit stiff. If available, Moxa is applied for 10 – 15 minutes.

SP 10, Xue Hai (血海)

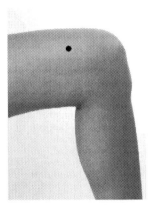

Location: With the knee flexed, 2 cun above the superior medial border of the patella.

How to find the pressure point: Sitting with knees at ninety degrees, palms on the knees. The thumb and the other four fingers are at a forty-five-degree angle, and the tip of the thumb is the points.

Benefits: Cools the Blood. Invigorates the Blood circulation. Enables the transformation of blood into energy. Regulates menstruation.

Indications: Urticaria. Eczema. Erysipelas. Herpes Zoster. Irregular menstruation, painful. Allergies.

Method of Application: With the thumb tip pressing the points for 3-5 minutes. The massage can be a bit stiff. If available, Moxa is applied for 10 – 15 minutes.

Note: If the massage is done before 11 am, it will be more effective.

SP 21, Da Bao (大包)

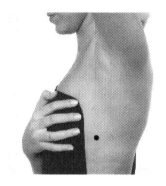

Location: On the mid-axillary line in the 6th intercostal space.

How to find the pressure point: Draw a line from the midpoint along the underarm. Draw other lines across from the nipple, to intersect with the midline, the gap between the two ribs is the point.

Benefits: The special effect for women is the protection of the chest health and shape. Due to its close proximity to the armpits, it has a protective effect on the lymphatic system. It has positive effects on breathing. It is beneficial to decrease general pain. Keeps the whole body in balance. Supports the immune system. Invigorates the Blood. Benefits the tendons. Regulates the Qi of the chest. Supports lactation. Keeps blood sugar in balance.

Indications: Pain throughout the body. Fibromyalgia. Sagging and pain in the limbs. Weak joints. Cough. Shortness of breath. Pain in the chest and ribs.

Method of Application: Put two palms on both sides of the chest and massage for 12-18 times.

Caution: Avoid Hard pressure.

Points of the Heart meridian

HT 3, Shao Hai (少海)

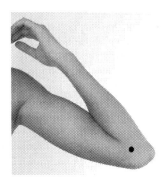

Location: With the elbow flexed, between the ulnar end of the cubital crease and the medial epicondyle of the humerus.

How to find the pressure point: Inside the elbow, at the end of the line formed when the elbow is bent, the gap between muscle and bone is the point.

Benefits: Unblocks and opens the meridian. Calms the Mind. Clears overheating from the body. Protects the heart from damage caused by excessive emotional factors. It is highly effective in reducing or eliminating fear.

Indications: Fullness in the chest. Pain in the armpit. Elbow pain. Manic behaviour. Anxiety. Soothes, gives a feeling of lightness. Reduces or eliminates fear.

Method of Application: First, by rubbing the point on the left side with the right thumb, 12 - 18 times massage, then with the help of the left thumb, the same procedure is performed on the right arm. If available, Moxa is applied for 10 – 15 minutes.

Points of the Small Intestine Meridian

SI 3, Hou Xi (后溪)

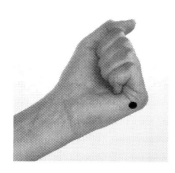

Location: On the ulnar end of the distal palmar crease, proximal to the 5th metacarpophalangeal joint, at the end of the transverse crease and the junction of the red and white skin.

How to find the pressure point: When the fist is half-closed, the protrusion at the end of the line extending from the palm to the side of the little finger is the point we are looking for.

Benefits: The special effect is for people who work hard at the computer. If we apply pressure to this point once an hour at work, it will rest your brain, which helps you work more efficiently. Also, it can rest your hands and arms, preventing shoulder pain. Other benefits are: regulating the Du Mai (Governing Vessel). Supports tendons. Clears the mind. Calms the soul, gives a feeling of freshness.

Indications: Occipital Headache. Dizziness. Vertigo. Stiff neck. Difficulty turning the neck. Pain in the upper back, shoulder, scapula and lumbar region. Pain and swelling of the eyes. Depression.

Method of Application: With Thumb, 12 - 18 times massage from little finger to wrist. If available, Moxa is applied for 10 – 15 minutes.

SI 6, Yang Lao (养老)

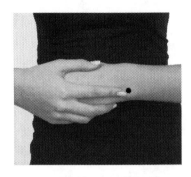

Location: Dorsal to the head of the ulna in the bony cleft on the radial side of the styloid process, found with the palm facing the chest.

How to find the pressure point: First hold the wrist with the palm facing down, put your index finger over the ulna bones protrusion, then turn the wrist towards yourself, the point where the fingertip comes from is the point we are looking for is in the middle on top of the wrist.

Benefits: Especially for a high-quality lifestyle in old age, delays various complaints that occur with age. Reduces fatigue, reduces pain. Benefits of the tendons. Especially eye problems that occur with senility. Good for arm, wrist, shoulder pain. It provides a positive effect for a more peaceful old age.

Indications: Blurred vision. Eye pain. *Bi* syndrome (Painful obstruction) in the shoulder, arm, elbow, wrist and feet. Swelling in the elbow. Stiffness of tendons.

Method of Application: Massages 3 minutes with the tip of the right index finger, pressing the point on the left wrist, then changing hands. If available, moxa is applied for 10 minutes once a week for both sides.

SI 11, Tian Zong (天宗)

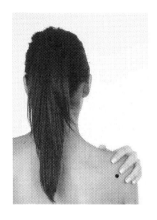

Location: On the scapula, in a depression 1/3 of the way from the midpoint of the inferior border of the scapular spine to the apex of the scapula.

How to find the pressure point: Put your hand on the shoulder, hold the thumb to show the neck. The point we are looking for is where the middle finger touches.

Benefits: Benefits of the breast's health. Strengthens the Yang energy. Especially relieves excessive arm fatigue. It is useful for protecting the shoulder area and removing complaints. Reduces the tension of the neck muscles.

Indications: Cricked neck. Frozen shoulder. Pain in the shoulder and scapula. Pain in the chest and side of the ribs. Swelling and pain in the breasts. Poor lactation.

Method of Application: First the left, then the right, With the thumb, do pressure masage from the outside to the inside, lower to upper on the point 12 to 18 times.

Note: It is important to drink a cup of water if you are using it for trouble in the gut and breast. If you use the shoulder or neck, the shoulder should keep warm and protected from the wind.

If available, Moxa is applied for 10 – 15 minutes.

SI 19, Ting Gong (听宫)

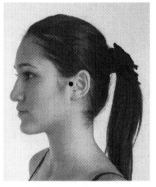

Location: In the anterior depression of the tragus. More easily found when you open your mouth.

How to find the pressure point: Where the jaw meets the ear, when you open your mouth, the middle of the pit formed is the point we are looking for.

Benefits: Keeps the ear function in balance, provides the hot cold setting on the face, prevents and delays the jaw sag.

Indications: Tinnitus. Pain or itching in the ear. Dizziness. Tinnitus.

Method of Application: With the middle finger, do pressure massage 12 - 18 times every day.

Caution: Avoid hard pressure.

Points of the Bladder Meridian

BL 1, Jing Ming (睛明)

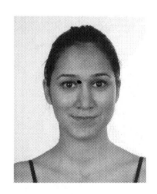

Location: On the face, in the depression superior to the inner canthus.

How to find the pressure point: On the nose side of the eye, it is the space in the inner corner of the eye (canthus).

Benefits: It helps to maintain eye function in a balanced way. Supports the secretion of the lacrimal gland. Controls the rise of the Yin Qi and Yang Qi to the eyes. It affects the function of tissues and organs in places where the bladder passes through the meridian.

Indications: Ocular dysfunction. Lacrimation (Tears). Dry eyes. Headache. Redness, swelling, pain, and itching in the eyes.

Method of Application: Put two elbows on the table, the thumbs looking up and place on the point, fix the

remaining fingers on the forehead, apply gentle pressure on the spot with the thumb 12 - 18 times.

Caution: Hands should be spotless and hard pressure should be avoided.

BL 11, Da Zhu (大杼)

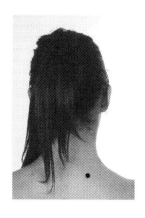

Location: On the upper back, at the midline and two fingers of the first vertebra (T1).

How to find the pressure point: First, the neck leans forward, find seventh neck spine protrusion (Spinous process), from which move down one vertebra, draw a horizontal line at the same level, two fingers from the midline. The point we are looking for is on the outer edge of the finger.

Benefits: Nourishes the Blood. By sending cool energy to the head side, it reduces boredom, gives a feeling of peace. Controls Liver Yang energy. Strengthens bones.

Indications: Anemia. Rhinitis. Low immunity. Stiff neck and back. Cough. Chest fullness. Breathlessness. Muscle and bone pain. Cough. Back pain. Stiff neck. Asthma.

Method of Application: It is done with the help of someone. Sit down, arms fixed on the table, or lie down face down. With the help of two thumbs, massage performed by rubbing the spot on both sides at the same time. Massage should be carried out together with breathing. When breathing, fingers relaxed, when breathing out, exert pressure for 12-18 times.

If available, Moxa is applied for 5-6 minutes.

BL 40, Wei Zhong (委中)

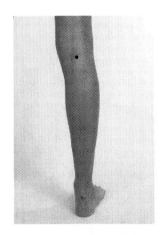

Location: The midpoint of the transverse crease of the popliteal fossa, between the tendons of biceps femoris and semitendinosus.

How to find the pressure point: In the midline (popliteal crease) behind the knee.

Benefits: The negative energy in the bladder meridian is collected here, cleaned, then sent down. There are nerves, vessels and lymph nodes passing through this region, which means there may be more negative energy around here which needs to be cleared to improve health and energy flow.

Indications: An effective acupoint for lower back pain. Improve lactation. Sciatica. Knee pain. Fever. Aversion to cold. Sweating. Headache. Heaviness.

Method of Application: Sit down and extend the legs in a chair, four fingers are rubbed from the inside to outside and from down to up for 2-3 minutes. Because of the detox effect, this massage can be applied once a week for a healthy life. I also use this point for cellulite treatment.

Caution: Hard impacts should be avoided. Drink one cup of warm water before and after the application. Do not apply moxa.

Note: *I would like to share an experience with these acupoints: My teacher told me "We can't use moxa for this point". I wanted to learn the reason. One day, I applied moxa for these acupoints. That night my fever was up to 39 degrees. I applied physical cooling and acupuncture. A few minutes later, I fell into a deep sleep, as if I was unconscious. When I woke up in the morning, I was feeling more vigorous than ever. It was an incredible experience for me. This showed me that moxa is definitely not recommended for this point.*

BL 57, Cheng Shan (承山)

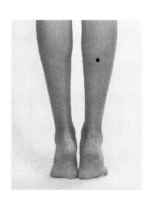

Location: 8 cun below BL 40 in a pointed depression below the gastrocnemius when leg is outstretched, or heel is lifted.

How to find the pressure point: In the middle of the calf. Stand on your toes, the muscle in the calf is pulled up, a triangular pit will be seen under the pulled muscle. The point we are looking for is the top space of the triangle.

Benefits: It nourishes the muscles in the region, strengthens the immune system. It is useful in disposing of body waste. Supports athletes to have strong muscles. Relaxes the tendons. Treats haemorrhoids.

Indications: Low back pain. Sciatica. Tension on the tendons. knee weakness. Leg muscles cramp and pain. Constipation

Method of Application: Sit comfortably, pull one leg towards you and place it on the other leg. Breathe deeply, press the point with two thumbs while exhaling, repeat this procedure 12-18 times. If available, Moxa is applied for 10 – 15 minutes.

Caution: After the massage, keep the area warm. If you feel pain if when you do the massage, avoid hard pressure. Apply a little more pressure when pain reduces.

BL 60, Kun Lun (昆仑)

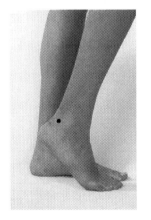

Location: In a depression between the tip of the external malleolus and the Achilles tendon.

How to find the pressure point: The gap between the ankle bone and the tendon.

Benefits: Strengthens the back. Invigorates the Blood.

Indications: Headache. Eye fatigue. Lower back pain. Sciatica. Abdominal distension/bloating. High blood pressure. Cold feet and heel spur. It also strengthens body resistance.

Method of Application: The thumb is placed on the point, breathing deeply, pressing the point while exhaling.

Recommend it to massage with the help of massage oil. If available, Moxa is applied for 10 – 15 minutes.

When talking about Kunlun points, I want to add a little bit about The Kunlun Mountain. It is located within the borders of China's Xinjiang Uighur Autonomous Region. This is the homeland of the Tulip. In this area there are Uygur, Kazak, Uzbek, Kyrgyz and Tatar people living there.

From this comparison, we can understand clearly how important these points are. Maybe Kunlun Mountains are the place where this point was found? Maybe the points come from old Turkic people's culture?

Points of the Kidney Meridian

KI 1, Yong Quan (涌泉)

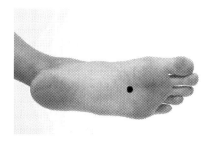

Location: On the sole of the foot, between the 2nd and 3rd metatarsal bones at the crease made by toe flexion at the metatarsophalangeal joints.

How to find the pressure point: Pin down all the toes. A pit is formed under the base, at the front. Press your thumb into the pit, then open the foot. The point where the thumb is held.

Benefits: It is one of the most important points. Makes you fit, energetic, peaceful, powerful. Calms the Mind. It exchanges energy with the earth. Protection from disease has a positive effect on healthy life. The foot is like the root of the tree, if the root is intact, the tree is strong.

Indications: Stress, fatigue, insomnia, dizziness. Menopausal complaints. Cold feet. Sweat. Sexual problems. Cramps. Night sweating. Anxiety. Poor memory. Fear. Fury. Manic behaviour. With moxa it is particularly effective for cold feet and cold lower limbs.

Note: This point is one of the lifeguard points (First aid point) for heat stroke or shock.

Method of Application: First use hot water to soak your feet, dry, then press with your thumb until local soreness is relieved.

If available, Moxa is applied for 10 – 15 minutes.

Caution: Not used in pregnant women or infants.

KI 3, Tai Xi (太溪)

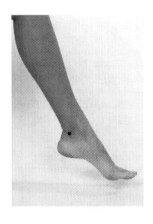

Location: In depression midway between the tip of the medial malleolus and the attachment of the Achilles tendon.

How to find the pressure point: In the depression between the internal malleolus and the tendon.

Benefits: It is a point that acupuncture doctors like to use, because it can get good results fast. Tonifies Kidney Yin and Yang energy. Calms the Mind. Strengthens the lower back and knees. Regulates the uterus.

Indications: Headache. Toothache. Fatigue. Forgetfulness. Ankle and wrist cold. It is also frequently used to reduce menstrual pain. Heel spur and sciatica. It also strengthens body resistance. Weakness. Cold and weak knees. Night sweating. Hot palms.

Breathlessness. Impotence. Premature ejaculation. Irregular menstruation.

Method of Application: Before going to bed every night, press with your thumb 12-18 times. If available, Moxa is applied for 10 – 15 minutes.

KI 6, Zhao Hai (照海)

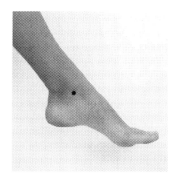

Location: 1 cun below the apex of the medial malleolus.

How to find the pressure point: Pushing vertically downward from the inner ankle till you feel a pit. That is the point we are looking for.

Benefits: Calms the Mind. Regulates uterus and menstruation. Benefits eyes and throat. It keeps kidney function in balance so that our life energy is always strong and flowing.

Indications: Night sweating. Backache. Insomnia. Sadness. Fear. Nightmares. Genital pruritus(itching). Pain, stress, and strain of the internal muscles of the legs. Cramp in the lower limb. Dry cough. Irregular and painful menstruation. Navel pain postpartum. Beriberi (Athlete's foot).

Method of Application: From the points, up to down press with your thumb 12-18 times. If available, Moxa is applied for 10 – 15 minutes.

KI 27, Shu Fu (俞府)

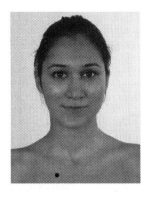

Location: 2 cun lateral to the midline, in the inferior margin of the clavicle.

How to find the pressure point: Under the bottom of the collarbone, move your finger from outside to inside, the place where the gap ends is the point.

Benefits: It is the immune booster point. Breath effect positively, provides body heat balance.

Indications: Cough. Difficult breathing. Asthma. Shortness of breath. Pain and fullness in the chest. Heavy sweating, cold feet, low body resistance, anorexia.

Method of Application: Tap with your fingers 3 minutes.

Points of the Pericardium Meridian

PC 6, Nei Guan (内关)

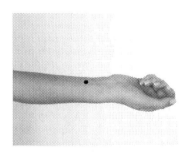

Location: 2 cun above the wrist crease between the tendons of palmaris longus and flexor carpi radialis.

How to find the pressure point: Three horizontal fingers up from the inner wrist.

Benefits: This is a very important point in our body. It is known to be effective in water metabolism. It has the effect of protecting the heart. It is believed to be one of the most important protective acupoints in the body, especially the heart. It makes a positive impact on the soul.

Indications: Pain and distention in the chest and abdomen. Nausea. Reflux. Vomiting. Hiccup. Belching. Irregular and painful menstruation. Insomnia. Manic behaviour. Poor memory. Anxiety. Fear. Sadness. Depression. PMS (Premenstrual syndrome).

Method of Application: Left thumb press the right the acupoint 18-30 times. Then exchange hands to the opposite side to do the same thing. If available, Moxa is applied for 5-10 minutes.

Points of the Triple Burner Meridian

SJ 3, Zhong Zhu (中渚)

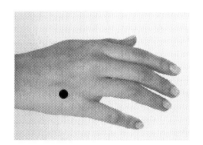

Location: With fist clenched, on the dorsum of the hand between the 4th and 5th metacarpal bones in the depression proximal to the 4th metacarpophalangeal joint.

How to find the pressure point: Back of the hand, the pit of fourth and fifth knuckles.

Benefits: Benefits ears. Controls Liver function. It has a positive effect on the energy flow in the three-burner meridians. Acts as chief for coordinated work of organs. In particular, stimulating to this point benefits people with ear problems.

Indications: Itching and redness in the face. Fever. Tinnitus. Earache and new hearing loss. Temporal head pain. Inability to flex or extend the fingers. It is beneficial in tinnitus and hearing loss due to side effects of medication. It is effective in providing heat balance.

Method of Application: Massage from bottom to top with your thumb 12-18 times. If available, Moxa is applied for 10 – 15 minutes.

SJ 5, Wai Guan (外关)

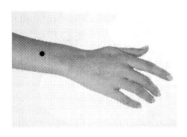

Location: 2 cun proximal to the dorsal wrist crease between the radius and ulna, close to the radial bone.

How to find the pressure point: Hold your hand with the palm facing down, three fingers on the back of the hand, in the middle of the radius with Ulna.

Benefits: Clears Heat from the head. Controls Liver Yang energy. Remove channel obstruction. Benefits ears. It is especially effective in hand finger problems. Helps for wrist pain. Increases resistance to disease.

Indications: Restricted bending and stretching of the arm. Pain in the fingers. Hand tremors. Fever. Chill. Aversion to cold. Bitter taste. Swelling and pain in the ear. Mumps. Unilateral headache. Pain in neck, shoulder, arm, elbow, wrist and fingers.

Method of Application: 12 - 18 times by pressing or rubbing with the thumb. The direction of the massage should be from the wrist to the arm direction. If available, Moxa is applied for 10 – 15 minutes.

Points of the Gallbladder Meridian

GB 31, Feng Shi (风市)

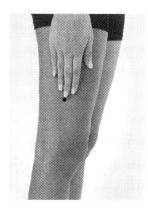

Location: In the lateral thigh. With the arm across the body, the point lies by the tip of the middle finger.

How to find the pressure point: Standing, arms hanging down, palms straight, the points at the tip of the middle finger.

Benefits: It affects the secretion of bile fluid positively. Supports fat metabolism. Prevents cellulite formation. Strengthens the immune system. Helps people to be determined. Good for insomnia. Good for leg muscle pain.

Indications: Herpes zoster. Itching. Urticaria. Paralysis, atrophy and leg pain. Weakness in the legs. Leg numbness and feeling cold, cellulite, weight loss.

Method of Application: Sit down and tap 30 times with a loose fist. If working for cellulite, weight loss, can massage more as you like, but not more then 10 minutes.

Note: It is important to drink a glass of warm water before and after the massage. If possible, do this process in the morning. If available, Moxa is applied for 10 – 15 minutes.

GB34, Yang Ling Quan (阳陵泉)

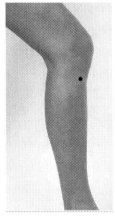

Location: In a depression anterior and inferior to the head of the fibula.

How to find the pressure point: Slightly curved the knee, External knee joint. The lower part of the tab of the fibula.

Benefits: Balances bile secretion. Supports the digestive system. Reduces the damage to the liver, so protects the liver. Benefits of the tendons. Helps to lose weight.

Indications: Irritability. Bad temper. Depression. Sigh. Bitter taste. Difficulty digesting fat. Feeling heaviness on the body. Tension on the tendons. Muscle stiffness. Cramp.

Method of Application: With the thumb pressing the points for 3-5 minutes. If available, Moxa is applied for 10 – 15 minutes.

GB 44, Zu Qiao Yin (足窍阴)

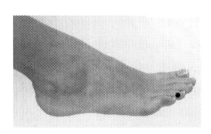

Location: 0.1 cun posterior to the corner of the nail on the lateral side of the 4th toenail.

How to find the pressure point: On the fourth toe, on the side of the nail, on the little toe side.

Benefits: Detoxifies. Controls Liver Yang energy. Brightens the eyes. Calms the Mind.

Indications: Various headaches (especially migraines around the eyes). Dizziness; Tinnitus; Insomnia. Nightmares; Excessive dreaming. Anxiety.

Method of Application: With the thumb tip 12-18 times pressing the points. It can be applied by putting wheat grain on the points when you massage, to make more feeling. If available, Moxa is applied for 10 – 15 minutes.

Points of the Liver Meridian

LR 3, Tai Chong (太冲)

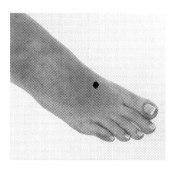

Location: On the dorsum of the foot in a depression distal to the junctions of the 1ˢᵗ and 2ⁿᵈ metatarsal bones.

How to find the pressure point: On the top surface of the foot. Use your thumb to push in between the first and second toe gaps, move the thumb along until it stops. These are the points.

Benefits: These are my favourite points that I almost use for everyone. Due to its detoxification effect, it is a useful point for the strength of the body. Controls Liver Yang energy. Reduces anger. Regulates menstruation. Calms the Mind. Resolves spasms.

Indications: Liver diseases and excessive alcohol intake. These points are effective in improving even damaged liver functions. Headaches. Dizziness; Blurred vision. Numbness of the head. Irritability. Anger. Insomnia. Constipation. Genital pain. Urinary difficulty. Irregular and painful menstruation and Cramps.

Method of Application: Choose a convenient time of day. Sit down in a comfortable position. Pull one bent leg towards you, massage the point with your thumb back and forth 12-18 times. You may have felt that this point is very painful or feels sore when you massage, which means we are exhausting our liver and need to take care of it. As the massage continues, the feeling of pain will be reduced day by day.

If available, Moxa is applied for 10 – 15 minutes.

Note: It is important to drink a glass of warm water and deep breathing when we massage. If you want to apply a cure to yourself, you need to avoid the animal food and go to bed early by following the working hours of the liver.

Caution: It is forbidden to use in pregnant women.

Points of the Ren Meridian

RN 3, Zhong Ji (中极)

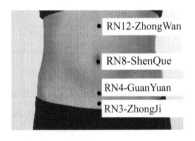

RN12-ZhongWan
RN8-ShenQue
RN4-GuanYuan
RN3-ZhongJi

Location: 4 cun below the navel. 1 cun above CV2 (pubic symphysis).

How to find the pressure point: In the lower abdomen, on the front midline, the front midline, from the centre of the navel, down five fingers.

Benefits: It sends Qi into your body without stopping. Strengthens the Kidney. Benefits the Uterus. Regulates menstruation.

Indications: Itching, pain, discharge and swelling of the genitals. Frequent urination. Cystitis. Irregular menstruation. Weak knees. Prostate problems. Provide postnatal balance.

Method of Application: Warm the palm, two palms in a row and place them on the point. Focusing on the acupoint, 5-10 minutes of deep breathing. If you continue this exercise, after a few days, you will be able to feel warmth in the whole body. That tells you the massage is working. You can also massage the point at the same time. While exhaling, you can do the finger pressing massage 12-18 times, relax your hands while inhaling.

If available, Moxa is applied for 10 – 15 minutes.

Caution: In children, severe pressure should be avoided. Not used on pregnant women.

RN 4, Guan Yuan (关元)

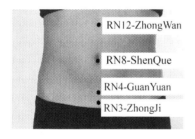

RN12-ZhongWan

RN8-ShenQue

RN4-GuanYuan

RN3-ZhongJi

Location: 2 cun above CV2 pubic symphysis.

How to find the pressure point: In the lower abdomen, on the front midline, from the centre of the navel, down four fingers.

Benefits: Nourishes the Blood. Strengthens the Kidney. It always makes you energetic. Benefits of the Bladder and the uterus. Regulates menstruation. Regulates Small Intestine.

Indications: Fear; Insomnia; Anxiety; Low back pain; Weak knees; Cold sensation in the back; Impotence; Cold sensation in the vagina; Painful urination. Women with menopause, menstrual problems, urinary incontinence is a useful acupoint.

Method of Application: Warm the palm, two palms in a row and placed on the point. Focusing the point, 5-10 minutes of deep breathing. If you continue this exercise, after a few days, you can feel warmth in the whole body. You also can massage the point at the same time. While exhaling, you can do the finger pressing massage 12-18 times, relax your hands while inhaling. Moxa can be applied for 10-15 minutes.

Caution: In children, severe pressure should be avoided. Not to be used on pregnant women.

RN 8, Shen Que (神阙)

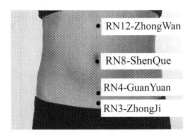

RN12-ZhongWan

RN8-ShenQue

RN4-GuanYuan

RN3-ZhongJi

Location: In the centre of the navel.

How to find the pressure point: See above

Benefits: Awakens the yang energy again. Helps us feel more energetic. Strengthens the Spleen.

Indications: This point is effective in babies crying because of gas pain. Feeling weakness, Nocturnal enuresis (bed-wetting).

Adding: We know that the baby in the uterus is fed nutrients and oxygen from the placenta. When the baby is born, the umbilical cord is cut off, and the baby starts to breathe through the lungs.

Chinese Medicine believes that natural breathability is hidden in the belly after the withdrawal of the umbilical cord and that this function can be re-stimulated if proper breathing is performed.

If this feature is re-stimulated, an energy tank is formed in our body and the energy flow in the human body is naturally rebalanced. Thus, it can be seen that human beings can be healthier and stronger through breathing exercises. As we age, our fixed energy is reduced and the energy stimulated supports the lack of Yang energy. This point is believed to carry the personality or character due to the mother's umbilical cord, which was previously connected.

Method of Application:

The palm is heated by rubbing against each other, the right hand are placed on top of the belly, lie on your back, your right hand on your navel, and a small cushion under your left elbow, and then take a deep breath for five minutes.

The desired effect is the spread of a slight temperature in the whole body. The breathing exercises can be done five days a week or every day.

If used for children, only use the warmed hands, no turning motion is made.

Considerations: Hands should be absolutely clean, no nail contact, no irritation to the area. The body should be kept warm after the application. Not to be used on pregnant women.

RN 12, Zhong Wan (中脘)

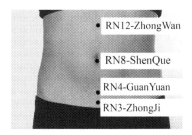

RN12-ZhongWan

RN8-ShenQue

RN4-GuanYuan

RN3-ZhongJi

Location: On the midline, 4 cun superior to the umbilicus.

How to find the pressure point: In the upper abdomen, on the front midline, from the centre of the navel, upward for five fingers.

Benefits: Supports the function of the Stomach and Spleen. Calms the Mind. Gives a feeling of peace.

Indications: Tiredness. Poor appetite. Pain in the stomach (stomach-ache). Digestion is difficult. Stomach pain. Abdominal distention. Gastric reflux and acid regurgitation. Vomiting. Diarrhea, Anxiety. Fear. Impatience.

Method of Application: Warm your palm, lie on your back, place the right palm on the point. Leave the left palm open, focus on the point and take a deep breath for 8-10 minutes. If you want to massage here, only use rubbing techniques.

If available, Moxa is applied for 10 – 15 minutes.

Caution: Do not do this exercise when you are full. This exercise should be done fondly, stroking, and avoiding hard pressing.

RN 17, Dan Zhong (膻中)

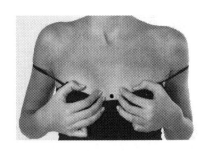

Location: In a depression on the midline, on the sternum, level with the 4th intercostal space.

How to find the pressure point: Lie down on your back, pull a line that connects the two nipples. The intersection with the middle line is the point we are looking for.

Benefits: Reduces distress, gives happiness, keeps the exchange of love in balance. Helps to defeat fear, reduces unrest. Promotes initial lactation. Improves immunity.

Indications: Fatigue, Low immunity. Spontaneous sweating. Chest pain. Breathlessness. Fullness or tightness in the chest. Psychological problems. For example: insomnia, unhappiness, feeling of fatigue, crying a lot or can't cry; Depression; Anxiety.

Method of Application: Sit cross-legged, or lie on your back, right hands put on the acupoint, breathing deeply and slowly. When breathing out, turn your hand clockwise. Do this exercise 8-12 times.

Moxa is **not** applied.

Caution: Avoid Hard pressure. Do not apply if there is heart disease, or after heart surgery.

RN 23, Lian Quan (廉泉)

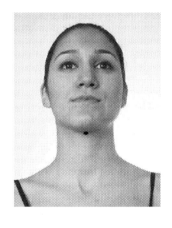

Location: In the anterior midline where the neck meets the head.

How to find the pressure point: In the middle line, above the throat bulge, between the neck and jowl.

Benefits: Support the speech problems, vocal cords and hoarseness. Bring self-confidence. Strengthens the immune system. It delays the formation of the dewlap (jowl).

Indications: Protect the vocal cords, good for hoarseness, sudden loss of voice, and dry throat.

Meridian: Conception Vessel (Ren Mai)

Method of Application: Method one, massage: Sit comfortably, fix your elbow on the table. rub the two thumbs upwards from the bottom. Massage is done 12 - 18 times.

Method two, breathing Exercise: Sit comfortably, close your mouth and breathe through the nose and feel the air through the throat. When breathing out, lightly open your mouth and let the air out. Do this slowly, you will hear the sound of the larynx when you do it right.

Note: For the second method, it is useful to get help from a professional.

Caution: Do not apply hard pressure.

RN 24, Cheng Jiang (承浆)

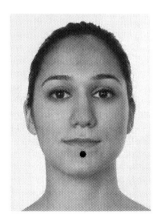

Location: In the midline, in the depression below the lower lip.

How to find the pressure point: Middle of lip and chin, on the middle line.

Benefits: Support for the secretion of saliva. Gives a feeling of satiety;

Indications: Facial swelling, numbness and pain. Gum inflammation and bleeding. Mouth and tongue wound. Facial paralysis

Method of Application: Put your elbow on the table, secure your chin with two thumbs. Then massage 3-5 minutes by placing two index fingers on top of each other underneath the chin. If you want to gain a feeling of fullness, do the massage counter clockwise. If you do this exercise while drinking a glass of warm water half an hour before a meal, you will see that you can't eat much. If you want to stimulate your appetite, you can do the same massage, but the direction will be counter clockwise.

Points of the Du Meridian

DU 4, Ming Men (命门)

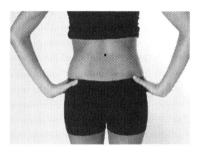

Location: Below L2 (2nd Lumbar vertebra).

How to find the pressure point: Place two hands on both sides of the waist, create a horizontal line to the spine. The point is the intersection of the midline.

Benefit: Tonifies original (inborn, Vital) energy. Can keeps the body temperature and heat distribution in balance, strengthens the vital function and ensures that it works in balance. Strengthens the lower back. Clears the Mind (Shen).

Indications: Backache. Tinnitus. Cold lower back. Tiredness. Impotence. Dysmenorrhea. Depression. Lack of willpower. Mental confusion. Depression.

Method of Application: Put your right hand in this area, do the diaphragmatic breathing. Contract the diaphragm so that air enters to the bottom of the lungs. The abdomen expands but the chest does not rise. Keep it warm for 10 minutes. After a few days, you can feel the warmth in the spine.

Considerations: It is important to keep this area warm after the massage. When not kept warm, the amount of energy is considered to be reduced, the organs cannot be fed enough. If it continues for a long time, the DU meridian may cause its energy to block.

DU 12, Shen Chu (身柱)

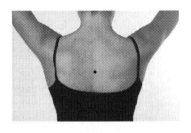

Location: On the midline below T3.

How to find the pressure point: Tilt your neck forward, in the spine line, you will see a mound in the back of the neck, that's the 7th spinous process. Countdown three vertebrae from here, and the space under the spine you find is the point we're looking for.

Benefit: It is useful for preventing colds in winter. It creates a strong, supported feeling. It is especially useful for raising children's body resistance. Reduces discomfort, lowers body temperature. It is useful for preventing colds in winter. Good for emotional problems. Just like when we are sad, we want someone to pat up our back. It creates a strong, supported feeling. Calms the Mind. Opens the windows of the soul.

Indications: Cough. Shortness of breath. Nightmare. Tiredness. Weak voice. Low immunity.

Method of Application: Rub very light touch on this point with a thumb or palm. The rotation direction is clockwise. Or the top-down friction applied on a straight line and the duration should be between 3 and 5 minutes.

Considerations: Avoid hard touch. Stroking is always the best move. We should keep the body warm after the massage.

DU 14, Da Zhui (大椎)

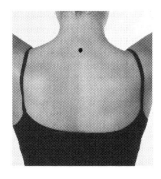

Location: On the midline, below C7 (7th cervical vertebra).

How to find the pressure point: Tilt your neck forward, in the spine line, you will see a mound in the back of the neck, that's the 7th spinous process, the space under the spine you find is the point we're looking for.

Benefits: Yang energy is powerful at this acupoint, so it can be effective in adjusting the body temperature. Soothes hot flushes. It regulates nutritive energy and defensive energy. Clears the Mind.

Indications: Fever. Feeling cold. Stiff neck. Depression. Tiredness. Menopause and complaints.

Method of Application: Self-application is difficult for this acupoint, so you will need someone's help. Sit comfortably, your helper stands on your left and puts the right hand on the area. Gently do friction massage for the area 12 - 18 times in the clockwise direction. Or just put your palm in the area, and warm it up for 10 minutes.

Considerations: Avoid hard movements, do not forget to drink plenty of water before and after work. No more than 5 minutes.

DU 20, Bai Hui (百会)

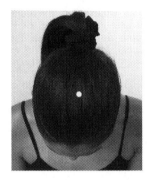

Location: It is at the top of the head, in the middle of the line connecting the two ears.

How to find the pressure point: At the top of the head, in the middle of the line connecting the two ears tip.

Benefits: Keeps Yang energy in balance and provides the integrity of the body. It is one of the most important acupoints. It helps to balance the energy required for brain function. Eliminates excessive stress, reduces anger, makes us more tolerant. It prevents forgetfulness and helps with concentration disturbance. Controls Liver Yang energy. Apparently, it's a great point to use for the continuity of body balance.

Indications: Headache, dizziness, poor memory, fear, restlessness, anxiety, tinnitus, sleep problems, depression, chronic fatigue, forgetfulness, impatience, hair loss, anger, smoking cessation, and weight loss Poor memory. Prolapse of internal organs. Haemorrhoids. We can also use it in angry, stressed, distressed, overjoyed times to relax.

Meridian: Governing Vessel (Du Mai)

Method of Application: Put the palm of your hand at the point of your head, taking a deep breath, massage the acupoint clockwise. The duration should be 2 - 3 minutes or 12 - 18 times. You can apply regularly twice a day. This massage can be done by lying down or sitting down.

Note: Massage should not be too hard. Should not be used in infants. The duration of the massage should not exceed 5 minutes.

DU 25, Su Liao – (素髎)

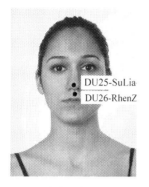

DU25-SuLia
DU26-RhenZ

Location: At the tip of the nose.

How to find the pressure point: At the tip of the nose.

Benefits: In clinical study, the effect of this point on re-stimulating and upgrading Yang energy is understood. That's why this point can raise the pulse and fallen blood pressure of a person in a state of shock and can correct breathing failure.

Indications: Cardiac Arrhythmia. Loss of consciousness. Rhinitis. Nasal secretion. Loss of smell.

Note: Moxa should not be used to this point. Suitable for adults, not for children.

DU 26, Ren Zhong – (人中)

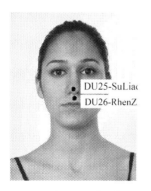

DU25-SuLiac
DU26-RhenZ

Location: In the first third of the distance between the nose and the upper lip.

How to find the pressure point: In the pit above the upper lip.

Benefits: This acupoint like Yang energy's command, strengthens and stimulates body energy. Because of its connection to the brain and the cortex, it has the power to revive the body and to stimulate consciousness. Calms the mind. It is like a human reset button.

Indications: Usually used in emergencies. Loss of consciousness. Stroke. Deviation of eye and mouth. Epilepsy crisis.

Method of Application: The middle finger is massaged 12-18 times with mild pressure. Finger pressing can be applied in emergency situations.

Note: Care should be taken not to damage the skin. Should not apply pressure for over 3 minutes.

Extra Points

As well as the main meridians described, and their related acupoints, there are extra meridians. Also there are acupoints that are not attached to a meridian. Furthermore, gentle probing can reveal locations on the body that are painful when touched. These are called Ashi points, so named because when they are touched the patients say "Ah. Shi", which means 'Ah. Yes'. Ashi points are the foundation of Extra points.

EX 2, Yin Tang – (印堂)

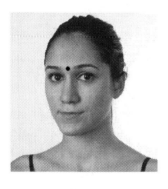

Location: In the middle of two eyebrows.

How to find the pressure point: As above

Benefits: Stress caused by fatigue, condensation disorder, forgetfulness, headache, anger, reluctance, low efficiency, fear, anxiety. Lack of determination. Fear. Nasal secretion, sinusitis. Increase smell.

Indications: Stress caused by fatigue, condensation disorder, forgetfulness, headache, anger, reluctance, low efficiency, fear, anxiety, insomnia or excessive sleep. Lack of determination. Fear. Nasal secretion. Sneezing.

Method of Application: With the index finger of both hands, slight pressure is applied on the sides 12 - 18 times from centre to two sides.

This point is frequently used in the China Turkish (Uyghur of Xinjiang) community for headache, and I knew that it was very effective when I was a child. When I was a little girl, my carer was a lady from a village of Hotan City in Xinjiang. She would massage the "Yin Tang" point between two eyebrows when she had a headache. I can remember her forehead between the two eyebrows was always red and purple. She always said: "This area reflects our character, heals our headache, and refreshes us."

She also said: "The red and purple colour here is the poison in our blood (we know it as a toxin today). She had never been to Mainland of China proper, but she knew this point as the tradition from her native village.

EX-HN-5, Tai Yang – (太阳)

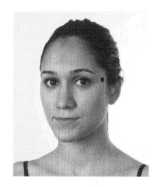

Location: In a depression 1 cun posterior to the midpoint between the lateral end of the eyebrow and the outer canthus.

How to find the pressure point: As above

Benefits: It supports and controls the liver Yang energy, gives people a sense of vigor, balances the excess energy, illuminates the eye, and helps to open the meridian network.

Indications: Brain fatigue, impaired concentration, forgetfulness, chronic fatigue, eye fatigue. Reduces blood pressure and reduces anger. Temporal headaches and Migraine. Dizziness. Blurred vision. Pain, swelling and redness in the eye.

Meridian: Extras

Method of Application: There is a special massage we can do at this point. Name is 'Return to spring'. Sit comfortably, put the palm to the two temples, all the fingers are held above the head, and only the palm is moved, first rubbing 6 - 12 times clockwise and then massaged in the opposite direction to the clock. You will feel your brain getting lighter before your work is finished. If you regularly massage this point every day, your brain will always be more efficient. There is also the effect of improving the quality of life by keeping brain function in balance.

Note Avoid hard pressure. If patients have high blood pressure they should work together with a practitioner with breathing exercises. Measure blood pressure before and after the massage.

EX-HN-6, Er Jian – (耳尖)

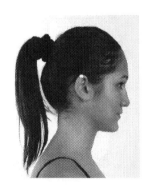

Location: At the apex of the ear.

How to find the pressure point: It is the highest place in the ear.

Benefits: It helps to reduce the excess heat (Yang energy) in the body and helps relax.

Indications: It is helpful in decreasing high blood pressure. It is very effective against high fever caused by swelling. It has a positive effect on mumps.

Method of Application: Place the elbow on the table, fasten the ear apex between the thumb and forefinger and rub it 12-18 times, apply gentle pressure if you feel pain.

Note: Should not use this point in people with low blood pressure.

EX-B-1, Ding Chuan – (定喘)

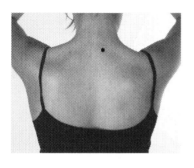

Location: 0.5 cun lateral to GV14 (Da Zhui)

How to find the pressure point: Head leans forward, find C7 (seventh neck spine) spinous process, horizontally one finger width beside this vertebra.

Benefits: Support the respiratory system.

Indications: Asthma. Breathlessness. Acute wheezing.

Method of Application: Sustained pressure and friction for 12-18 times, pressure can be a little strong.

Note: Stop after skin flushing. It is important to keep the body warm after massage.

EXUE-11, Shi Shuan – (十宣)

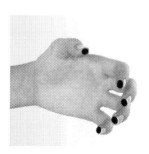

Location: At the tip of each finger.

How to find the pressure point: At the tip of each finger.

Benefits: Since fingertips are places where energy is concentrated, it makes a direct warning to our brain. It gives vitality to the body and distributes excess heat in the body. It has a positive effect on the blood circulation in the capillary.

Indications: Loss of consciousness, Hypertension, High fever, Anorexia, feeling cold, painful and numbness of the hand and fingers.

Method of Application: Tapping fingers on both hands for 3-5 minutes.

EX-UE-10, Si Feng – (四缝)

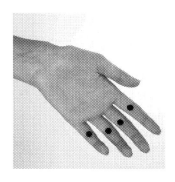

Location: Four points on each hand, on the palm side of the 2nd to 5th fingers and at the centre of the proximal interphalangeal joints.

How to find the pressure point: As above

Benefits: In particular, it facilitates digestion in children, helping to drain fullness and stagnant energy in the stomach.

Indication: Eating disorder in children, lack of appetite, vomiting.

Method of Application: 6-12 times massage is done with soft touches on serial points. If available, Moxa is applied for 10-15 minutes.

Note: Avoid harsh pressure in infants.

EM 30, Ba Xie – (八邪)

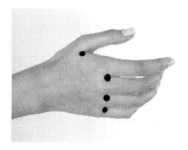

Location: On the web between each finger.

How to find the pressure point: When the fingers are close together, the points are at the end of the creases between each finger.

Benefits: Relaxes the tendons of the wrist, hand and fingers.

Indications: Relaxes the tendons of the wrist, hand and fingers. Pain, numbness, stiffness, swelling and spasm of the fingers. Headache, sore throat, anorexia, hot flushes, food poisoning, hand finger numbness and purification from toxins.

Method of Application: Two hands clasped together. 3 minutes of massage by applying pressure from where the fingers are clamped. Or rubs each individual finger. Should apply massage to each series of points 12-18 times.

Note: It is beneficial to drink plenty of water since it has a detox effect.

EX 32, Yao Tong Dian – (腰痛点)

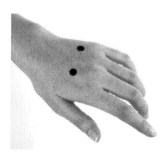

Location: Two points on the back of each hand, between the 2nd and 3rd and between the 4th and 5th metacarpal bones, approximately in the middle of the hand. Use the Hand of the side that is affected.

How to find the pressure point: On the dorsal aspect of the hand, glide with the palpating fingers in the grooves between the 2nd and 3rd and between the 4th and 5th metacarpal bones towards the wrist joint, until the fingers come to rest in the depressions just distal to the bases of the metacarpal bones.

Benefits: Treats the lower back.

Indications: Pain and tension in the lower back.

Method of Application: Use the hand of the side that is affected. Friction and sustained pressure for 3-5 minutes. Pressure can be strong. If you find the most painful points or nodules in the area, applying friction to the nodules becomes softer should be more effective. Moxa is applicable for 10-15 minutes for each of them.

Note: This method is used as an aid. Consult a qualified practitioner.

EX-LE-10, Ba Feng – (八风)

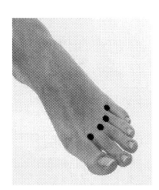

Location: Eight points on the dorsal surface of the foot located the webs between each of the toes.

How to find the pressure point: When the toes are closed together, the points are at the end of the creases between the toes.

Benefits: Relaxes the tendons. Expels dampness. Removes obstruction.

Indications: Restlessness throughout the body, low body resistance, purifying from toxins, in menstrual pain, menopause, hot flashes, cold feet, and spasms in the foot.

Method of Application: Open the toes, apply perpendicular pressure for 12-18 times. Friction also is effective. Moxa is applicable for 10-15 minutes for all the points.

Note: After the massage, should keep the foot warm and drink plenty of water.

Ex-UE-8, Lao Zhen Xue – (落枕穴)

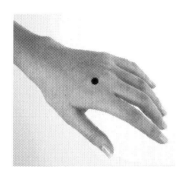

Location: On the dorsum of the hand, between the 2nd and 3rd metacarpals approximately 0.5 cm from the metacarpophalangeal joint centre.

How to find the pressure point: In the bone gap between the index finger and the middle finger on the back of the hand. Move your hand, the place where you feel the most pain is the point you are looking for.

Benefits: Treat the neck.

Indications: Stiff neck. Neck muscle fatigue (For example: working on the computer for a long time).

Method of Application: Use the Hand of the side that is affected. Applies perpendicular pressure 12 -18 times. Friction also is effective. To be more effective, you can slightly move your neck while massaging. Moxa is applied for 5-10 minutes for the points.

Note: After massage, the neck should be kept warm. Use the Hand of the side that is affected.

Gao Xue Ya Dian – (高血压点)

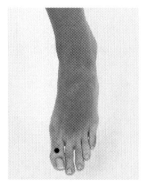

Location: It is in the middle of the deep line above the big toe.

How to find the pressure point: As above.

Working mechanism: It is a point that is used by believing that the pressure in the head comes out through the foot.

Benefits: When used regularly it will help to balance high blood pressure. It can add a positive effect to your drugs. Can also be applied when blood pressure suddenly rises.

Indications: High blood pressure

Method of Application: Applied horizontal pressure for 12-18 times. Friction also is effective.

Note: Remember to check blood pressure before and after the massage. Do not stop taking the medicine you are using.

CHAPTER 5
Signs, Symptoms and Solutions

Throughout our lives we are beset by little problems. Some of them are debilitating. Others are not so bad, merely irritations. Some are transient. Others are chronic. Some are symptoms of a more serious condition. Others are what they are and nothing more.

Here are some that yield well to manipulation of the acupoints that you learnt in the previous chapter.

Remember that the information here is for education. Individual situations will vary. These actions may give temporary relief. They are not a substitute for consulting a licensed health practitioner.

Abdominal distension

Abdominal distension occurs when substances, such as air (gas) or fluid, accumulate in the abdomen causing its expansion. It is typically a symptom of an underlying disease or dysfunction in the body. Sufferers often experience a sensation of fullness, abdominal pressure and possibly nausea, pain or cramping.

Bloating is most commonly because of a build-up of gas in the stomach, small intestine, or colon. A major cause of abnormal bloating is excessive eating and air swallowing. Women are more prone to bloating and often identify these symptoms during menstruation. Some individuals who develop distension may have poor motility of their intestines. Sometimes it may be due to hypersensitivity causing gut sensations. Giving medications, such as antidepressants and antispasmodics can contribute to reduced gut motility. Research has shown that swallowing air during eating or delayed emptying of the stomach from hyperacidity leads to bloating after a meal. Individuals who are constipated also complain of bloating. Other causes are often a digestive disorder or other organ diseases.

Bloating is not life-threatening. In most cases, we can handle bloating with simple home remedies and changes in lifestyle.

Acupoints Solution

ST 25, Tian Shu (天枢): Keeps bowel movement and large intestine energy in balance.

RN 8, Guan Yuan (关元): It strengthens the energy and makes the organism work in balance.

RN 12, Zhong Wan (中脘): Supports the stomach and spleen function, reduces swelling, provides airflow in the digestive system.

ST 36, Zu San Li (足三里): Maintains the balance of the digestive system, reduces stress and provides powerful energy.

DU 4, Ming Men (命门): Strengthens the body energy, reduces the feeling of nausea.

SP 6, Tai Chong (太冲): It is useful for easier disposal of blocked energy, helps to release gas.

Recommendations

> ➤ Eat less fat.
> ➤ Exercise strengthens the abdominal muscles.
> ➤ Learn the foods that cause you to bloat.
> ➤ Stay away from your late-night eating habits.
> ➤ Avoid overeating.

➢ Eat more slowly.

Aphonia (loss of sound or voice)

Aphonia means partial or complete loss of sound. Muteness or loss of voice is more common in singers, teachers and other occupations who do a lot of talking. Sometimes it can be caused by stress. Many risk factors can contribute to a voice disorder, including:

➢ Aging
➢ Alcohol use
➢ Allergies
➢ Gastroesophageal reflux disease (GERD)
➢ Illnesses, such as colds or upper respiratory infections
➢ Improper throat-clearing over a long time
➢ Neurological disorders
➢ Psychological stress
➢ Scarring from neck surgery or from trauma to the front of the neck
➢ Screaming
➢ Smoking
➢ Throat cancer
➢ Throat dehydration
➢ Thyroid problems

Voice misuse or overuse. Sometimes it can be caused by another disease. Treatment is usually done according to the cause.

Acupoints Solution

LU 10, Yu Ji 鱼际穴: This point helps the capillary in the region improve blood circulation. It has a direct positive effect on the vocal cords. Also provides sound protection.

RN 23, Lian Quan (廉泉): Reduces the vocal cords and surrounding inflammations. Important to note: Aphonia can sometimes be a harbinger of a more serious disease, so do not delay a visit to a doctor.

Back pain

Back pain is common and affects people of all ages. Usually it improves in a few days, weeks, or can continue for a lengthy period. Back pain is often associated with tension or stiffness. Several things can cause it, including your posture, a sudden movement or fall, an injury, or a medical condition. The pain relates to the way the bones, discs, tendons, muscles, and ligaments work together. Most people experience lower back pain at some point in their life.

TCM Overview

1. Kidney energy deficiency (Life energy deficiency): The symptoms of low back pain are mainly soreness, with weakness in the knees and legs. Excessive fatigue. Need to avoid excessive fatigue.
2. Blood stasis type: Blood slowing down, the back is mostly stinging, and the painful part is stable, and it is aggravated at night. Need to strengthen blood circulation.
3. Cold and damp type: The back is sore, often with a cold and heavy feeling. It intensifies in rainy weather. Need to warm meridians, dispelling cold and damp.

Damp heat type: Pain in the back, waist, and hips, a feeling of burning in the area. The treatment principle is to reduce heat in the area.

Acupoints solution

Li 11, Qu Qi (曲池): Reduces edema, relieves muscle tension, detoxifies.

SP 6, San Yin Jiao (三阴交): Balances spleen, kidney and liver meridians, reduces stress, makes you feel vigorous.

BL 40, Wei Zhong (委中): It is a special point for all kinds of lower back pain.

BL 60, Kun Lun (昆仑): Especially to help lower back pain and sciatica.

DU 4, Ming Men (命门): It especially helps for lower back pain caused by muscle fatigue. It is also beneficial for spine health.

KI 1, Yong Quan (涌泉): It helps to lower back pain, especially caused by excessive fatigue, raises life energy.

DU 14, Da Zhui (大椎): Reduces inflammation, helps general pain and positively affects the spine.

KI6, Zhao Hai (照海): Especially useful for lower back pain caused by excessive energy (overstrain) loss.

KI3, Tai Xi (太溪): Increase kidney energy and strengthens the lumbar region.

EX 32, Yao Tong Dian (腰痛点): It is a special experience for lower back pain and it really works.

Ashi Points (阿是穴): Find the sorest spot or area, warm the place using the palm of your hand.

We know Ashi as the point of most tenderness in TCM. It refers to a point or points of sensitivity or discomfort. Which should be chosen because of their responsive nature. Referring to the pain held in ones' tissues, muscles, and body. This pain can be physical or mental or emotional. Acupoints and meridians comprise a system of healing that penetrates beyond the surface and works with your body's energy to re-create balance within you. It works in obvious ways, and in more subtle ways.

Recommendation:

> ➢ Do exercises to strengthen the muscles of the abdomen and lumbar muscles, especially learn from a specialist before starting the exercises.
> ➢ Avoid carrying excess weight.
> ➢ Always keep the waist and soles of the feet warm.
> ➢ Avoid sudden movements.
> ➢ Always dry your back sweat.

Bed-wetting

Bed-wetting is involuntarily urinating during sleep beyond a reasonably appropriate age. Also called nocturnal enuresis. It's often just a normal part of a child's development. Before age 7 it isn't a concern.

TCM overview

According to TCM theory, this is due to insufficient kidney meridian energy, especially low *Yuan* Qi. In this case, the urine retention function at night of the kidney cannot be performed normally. The human body has an effective hormone to regulate water retention in our body called vasopressin or antidiuretic hormone (ADH). Inadequately secreted ADH reveals what they call "low kidney energy" in Chinese medicine. So, the treatment methods are carried out to strengthen the kidney meridian's energy and balance it.

Acupoints Solution

KI 1, Yong Quan (涌泉): it increases and strengthens the body's energy and warms the body.

RN 8, Guan Yuan (关元): Strengthens the energy in the region.

SP 6, San Yin Jiao (三阴交): Ensures that kidney and urinary tract function works in balance.

DU 20, Bai Hui (百会): Makes it easy to control.

RN 8, Shen Que (神阙): increase life energy, warms the body.

DU 4, Ming Men (命门): Increases body energy.

Recommendations:

➤ Keep the foot and waist warm.
➤ Wear 100% wool socks in winter.
➤ Do not drink excessive cold water.
➤ Do not sit in a cold place as cold stone.
➤ Consult your child's doctor if your child still wets the bed after age 7.
➤ Adults can do the exercise to strengthen the muscles in the region.

Note: The points may also be used in cases of incontinence in adults. But first you should learn from your doctor the cause of your illness, if you need treatment, do not neglect this

Chronic Fatigue Syndrome (CFS)

Chronic fatigue syndrome (CFS), is an illness that causes extreme fatigue; any other medical condition cannot explain that. If you have CFS you are likely to feel exhausted, even if you have not been active. Doctors do not yet understand the cause of CFS.

There's no single test to confirm a diagnosis of chronic fatigue syndrome. You may need a variety of medical tests to rule out other health problems that have similar symptoms. Treatment for chronic fatigue syndrome focuses on symptom relief.

Symptoms may include: Fatigue, loss of memory or concentration, sore throat, enlarged lymph nodes in your neck or armpits, unexplained muscle or joint pain, headaches, unrefreshing sleep, extreme exhaustion lasting over 24 hours after physical or mental exercise. TCM aims at reducing complaints, renewing, strengthening body energy, and improving immunity.

TCM overview

It is believed that CFS mainly relates to emotional factors. It is also related to poor eating habits and overwork. Long-term mental and psychological stress and overwork; causes the imbalance of meridians such as kidney, liver, heart, and spleen. Eventually caused body energy deficiency in the body. The principle of treatment is detoxification of the liver and improvement of kidney energy. Peace of mind, adjust mind and maintain spleen energy. Finally, strengthen the energy level of the whole body.

Acupoints Solution:

KI 1, Yong Quan (涌泉): Renewing, strengthening body energy, and improving immunity.

DU 20, Bai Hui (百会): It relieves the fatigue in the brain and gives a feeling of vitality.

SP 6, San Yin Jiao (三阴交): Purifies toxins and improve immunity.

ST 36, Zu San Li (足三里): Improve immunity, regulates blood circulation, provides energy.

DU 4, Ming Men (命门): Increases body energy.

LR 3, Tai Chong (太冲): Protect your eyes by regulating the liver.

Recommendations:

- ➢ Take care of your health, take time for yourself.
- ➢ Stop smoking.
- ➢ Keep your weight in balance.
- ➢ Take a shower with warm water every day and clean up your energy.
- ➢ Walk at least 3 times a week.
- ➢ Exercise breathing.
- ➢ Meditate.
- ➢ Take care not to eat excessively.
- ➢ Eat slowly while eating and reduce the load on the stomach.
- ➢ Try to wear cotton clothing.
- ➢ Listen to the music that revives you.

Consult with your doctor. Perhaps you should take the appropriate vitamin supplement.

Cold Hands and Feet

TCM Overview

According to TCM, the common reason for feeling cold is the lack of yang energy in the whole body. So, treatment generally is to enhance body energy.

Acupoints Solution

DU 4, Ming Men (命门): It warms the body by strengthening the life energy.

DU 14, Da Zhui (大椎): Balance the body temperature.

RN 4, Guan Yuan (关元): It awakens sleep energy and has a positive effect on blood circulation.

SP 6, San Yin Jiao (三阴交): It expels edema from the body, pushes cold energy out of the body.

KI 1, Yong Quan (涌泉): Increases energy and affects blood circulation positively.

LI 11, Qu Qi (曲池): Expels the cold air from the body.

Recommendations

> ➤ Consider clothing choices, wear cotton and wool clothing.
> ➤ Exercise every day. Exercise daily, including walking, to improve your blood circulation.
> ➤ Drink Cinnamon, Fresh ginger and Linden tea, can help you feel warm in the body.

Concentration Disorder and Forgetfulness

We all experience this situation from time to time. Human psychology directly affects this function. When we are worried, sad, undecided, restless, and exhausted, we experience forgetfulness and concentration problems. Old age or some diseases can cause the above complaints. Memory slips are aggravating, frustrating, and sometimes worrisome. Sometimes people can trigger fears of looming dementia or Alzheimer's disease.

There are six common treatable causes of forgetfulness.

1. Lack of sleep. Not getting enough sleep is perhaps the greatest unappreciated cause of forgetfulness.

2. Medications. Tranquilisers, antidepressants, some blood pressure drugs, and other medications can affect memory, usually by causing sedation or confusion.
3. Stress and anxiety. Both can interfere with attention and block the formation of new memories or the retrieval of old ones.
4. Depression. Common signs of depression include a stifling sadness, lack of drive, and a lessening of pleasure in things you ordinarily enjoy.
5. Alcohol. Drinking too much alcohol can interfere with short-term memory, even after the effects of alcohol have worn off.
6. Under-active thyroid. A faltering thyroid can affect memory (and disturb sleep and cause depression, both of which can be causes of forgetfulness).

TCM Overview

In classical Chinese philosophy, the belief is that the heart's function of managing emotions is imbalanced in this situation.

Acupoints Solution:

DU 20, Bai Hui (百会): It keeps the brain and body function in balance. Restores concentration.

EX 2, Yin Tang (印堂): Clarifies thoughts.

EX 3, Tai Yang (太阳): Rests the brain.

PC 6, Nei Guan (内关): It is the point that reduces or takes away the distress within us.

HT 7, Shen Men (神门): It rests our souls, gives us a peaceful feeling.

Recommendations:

> ➤ Maintain an active and orderly lifestyle.
> ➤ Learn to regulate yourself, think positively.
> ➤ Make it customary to note the location of your belongings.
> ➤ Take a walk outdoors.
> ➤ Meet your friends, chat.
> ➤ Practice breathing and listen to music.
> ➤ Solve riddles and do puzzles.
> ➤ Read and tell your friends what you have read.
> ➤ Enjoy getting more sleep.
> ➤ Take part in a stress reduction program.
> ➤ If memory lapses are affecting you, it's worth a conversation with your doctor to see if any reversible causes are at the root of the problem.

Constipation

Constipation can be annoying, and occasionally painful. It can usually be easily treated by making simple lifestyle changes.

Almost everyone gets constipated in their life at times. The colon can cause constipation by absorbing too much water from your food. This means your stools, which are produced at the end of the digestive process, get dry and hard, making them difficult to pass.

When people are not eating enough fibre, not drinking enough water, not exercising enough, pregnant, getting their period, using laxatives too much, taking certain medications such as painkillers or iron tablets, have a medical condition such as diabetes or a nerve disease, have a digestive problem, such as irritable bowel syndrome, diverticulitis or haemorrhoids, they can experience constipation.

TCM Overview

TCM sees constipation as a disease in its own right in Chinese medicine. Although there are many reasons, the main causes are energy deficiency or blockages that make the forward thrust of energy decrease. To compensate for such an imbalance is usually the first complaint in many diseases. The treatment principle is to strengthen Yang energy, to help energy moving. Acupoints Solutions

ST 25, Tian Shu (天枢): Keeps bowel movement and energy in balance.

LI 4, He Gu (合谷): Increase intestinal energy movement and provide intestinal water balance.

ST 36, Zu San Li (足三里): Maintains the balance of the digestive system, reduces stress and provides strong energy.

DU 20, Bai Hui (百会): Balance the whole body, reduces stress and headache caused by constipation, reduces the feeling of heaviness and fatigue.

Abdominal massage:

Stretch, curl your knees, clockwise massage your abdomen with sesame oil, between 30-50 times.

Do the massage every night before going to bed and go to the toilet the next morning. The best time is 5:00 -7:00 am. Continue this practice for 10-15 days. Do not use this massage when pregnant.

Recommendation:

➢ Eat plenty of fibre foods and fruits and vegetables;
➢ Drink enough water;
➢ Avoid excessive spice;
➢ Exercise regularly, strengthen your abdominal muscles;

> ➤ Move after sitting for a long time;
> ➤ Avoid excessive stress;
> ➤ Get to go to the toilet early in the morning;
> ➤ Perform regular abdominal massage.

Occasionally, constipation can be a sign of an underlying disease, such as bowel cancer. In such cases, there are likely to be other symptoms, such as a recent change in bowel habits, weight loss, anal bleeding or abdominal pain. If you have any of these symptoms, see your doctor.

Decreased Appetite

A decreased appetite occurs when you have a reduced desire to eat. The medical term for this is anorexia. A wide variety of conditions can cause your appetite to decrease. These range between mental and physical illnesses. It's important to find the reason behind your decreased appetite and treat it. Stress and excessive fatigue, sadness, depression, grieving, or anxiety, various psychological reasons, bad habits (alcohol, smoking, and other addictive substances), not to eat regularly, eating cold food continuously, disruption of sleep patterns, some drugs and diseases are the causes of loss of appetite. In most cases, your appetite will return to normal once to treat the underlying condition or reason.

TCM Overview

In Chinese medicine it is seen as external factors that disrupt our internal balance. The treatment is to get rid of the imbalance caused by external factors and to ensure internal balance.
Acupoints Solution

EX 28, Si Feng (四逢): It is especially effective for stimulating children's appetite.

LU 7, Lie Que (列缺): Used in adults, helps to enjoy the meal.

M–UE-1, Shi Shuan (十宣): Eliminates the blocked energy and gives you the desire to eat.

RN 8, Shen Que (神阙): Increasing the energy of life gives you the desire to eat.

ST 36, Zu San Li (足三里): Balance the digestive system maintains and gives the desire to eat.

EM 30, Ba Xie (八邪): It helps remove toxins from the body, activates the blocked energy and increases appetite.

Recommendations:

To maintain a normal life, one's appetite must remain normal. As well asusing the acupoints above, doing sports, hiking, avoiding stress and fatigue are also important things to do. If anorexia is caused by a disease, please see your doctor.

Eyestrain

Eyestrain occurs when after intense use, such as while driving long distances or looking at screens for a long time. It can be annoying, but it usually isn't a serious problem. Rest your eyes, or take other steps to reduce your eye discomfort, for quick relief. Sometimes, signs and symptoms of eyestrain can show an underlying eye problem that needs treatment.

TCM Overview

The liver is linked to the eyes. If the liver functions harmonically, the eyes can distinguish five colours and see very well. Among the internal organs, the liver and the eyes are most closely related. So, protecting the eyes usually begins with regulating the liver meridian. Acupoints Solution

ST 2, Si Bai (四白): It affects the blood circulation positively around the eyes, rests the eye muscles and gives a feeling of comfort.

BL1, Jing Ming (睛明): Gives the eye a sense of calmness, rests the eye muscles.

EX 2, Yin Tang –(印堂): Gives the eye a sense of calmness, rests the eye muscles.

EX 3, Tai Yang – (太阳): It rests the muscles of the eye, brightens the eye, regulates the energy flow in the region, reduces the feeling of bloating.

SP 6, Tai Chong (太冲): Protect your eyes by regulating the liver.

Recommendation:

➤ While working on the screen, keep your eyes away from the screen for 10 minutes after a maximum of two hours.
➤ Blinking is a natural eye massage. Blinking more can help rest your eyes.
➤ Close the eyes to rest.
➤ Try to look away from the screen every two hours.

Facial Skin and Beauty

We all want to have healthy-looking beautiful skin. So, if we learn a few acupoints, we can gain skin beauty naturally.

TCM Overview

The face is a place of the meeting of all the yang meridians. The six yang meridians connected on the head. It is the place where the whole-body yang energy reacts (or responds). It is also a part of mental concentration, facial expressions and demeanour are important contents of the expression and evidence of the spirit. The Inner Canon of the Yellow Emperor said that the five internal organs each have a different condition, and each has a specific relationship with the body. The face's colour is connected with the heart, the brightness of the skin depends on the lungs, the beauty of lip colour is about the spleen, the beauty of the nails is about the liver, the hair beauty's related to the kidney. So the skin's beauty should start from the entire body, especially from the five organs.

Acupoints solution:

Li 11, Qu Qi (曲池): Nourishes and revitalises skin. Purifies from toxins.

ST 4, Di Cang (地仓): Prevents the formation of lines around the lips. Gives colour for lips.

EX 2, Yin Tang (印堂): Gives the shine to face and delays formation of the line between the brow.

EX 3, Tai Yang (太阳): Nourishing skin around the eyes reduces tightness caused by stress.

RN 24, Lian Quan (廉泉): Delays the occurrence of tickling.

SP 6, San Yin Jiao (三阴交): Balances spleen, kidney and liver meridians, reduces stress and edema. It gives a clean look to the face.

SP 6, Tai Chong (太冲): Prevent age spots from forming. It softens the angry look.

Recommendations:

We need discipline to do skincare. You can work easily while applying a cream to your face in the morning or using a night cream after evening cleaning to massage your acupoints on the face. Drinking plenty of water and regular breathing practice will give you incredibly beautiful results.

➢ Clean your face in the morning and evening.
➢ Use sunscreen.
➢ Get rid of the habit of going to bed late.
➢ Take care of your water consumption.
➢ Eat less fried food, eat more fruits and vegetables.
➢ Try to laugh more.
➢ Be sure to wash your face after working on a computer.

Important: Massage on your face should never be rushed. The movements should be from bottom to top, from front to back. It is important to drink water before the massage.

Fear

Fear is a disturbing and negative feeling triggered by perception of threats in the face of uncertainty. Fear is a seemingly universal feeling. Everyone can experience various fears, consciously or unconsciously. A person who is in danger or scared, and as a result of this fear creates a reaction to escape (also known as a fight-or-flight response). Which in extreme cases of fear (horror and natural disasters) can be a freeze response or paralysis.

TCM overview

TCM believes that people have seven emotions including joy, anger, worry, anxiety, sadness, fear, and fright. The Chinese philosophy of life also believes the emotion of the kidney is fear. Some people have urinary incontinence when scared. Therefore, it focuses on the balancing of kidney energy to cure fear. And to help to provide inner peace.

Acupoints Solution

HT 7, Shen Men (神门): Calm the nerves, quiet down the mind.

HT 3, Shao Hai (少海): Especially effective for relieving fear.

DU 20, Bai Hui (百会): Makes it easy to control.

PC 6, Nei Guan (内关): Gives inner peace, regular the nervous system.

KI 1, Yong Quan (涌泉): It strengthens the kidney energy and warms the body.

DU 26, Ren Zhong (人中): It destroys panic, helps the Governor meridian and Ren meridian regain control. This is a point that saves lives.

Recommendations:

- ➢ Face your fears, talk about it.
- ➢ Do not be perfect, try to be yourself.
- ➢ Practice deep breathing every day and meditation.

Forgetfulness

Can't find your car keys? Forget your grocery list? Can't remember the name of the personal trainer you liked at the gym? You're not alone. Everyone forgets things occasionally. Still, memory loss is nothing to take lightly. Despising our body lowers kidney energy. The lack of energy cannot ensure regular functioning of the heart and spleen. Thus, the energy required to go to the heart and brain is insufficient, the brain cannot perform the function of remembering. The treatment is carried out by providing peace of mind, strengthening kidney energy, balancing brain function, and allowing energy to flow without clogging.

Acupoints Solution

1. **DU 20, Bai Hui** (百会): Gives peace of mind, improves forgetfulness, and stabilises brain function.
2. **HT 7, Shen Men** (神门): Improves forgetfulness by providing inner peace.
3. **PC 6, Nei Guan** (内关): It gives inner peace, does not allow the heart to "dissipate".
4. **KI 1, Yong Quan** (涌泉): It provides the best flow of energy, it helps the brain go to more energy.

Note: Although there are no guarantees for preventing memory loss or dementia, certain activities and memory exercises, such as solving puzzles or learning something new, might help.

Halitosis (Bad Breath)

Halitosis is the medical name for bad breath. The most common cause of bad breath is having tiny food particles trapped in your teeth and mouth. When the natural bacteria in your mouth break down these tiny bits of food, a foul-smelling gas is released. In Chinese Medicine it results from an imbalance of the internal organs, particularly of the digestive system. Unbalanced nutrition, late eating, eating heavy food, fever, excessive stress, constipation, wrong breathing, smoking, mouth, and teeth problems, not paying attention to the mouth is part of the causes of bad breath. Some medical conditions can also cause bad breath. Other factors causing bad breath include strong-flavoured foods, such as garlic and onion, and smoking. Although this does not appear to be a serious illness, it is often a negative impact on people's social relationships and self-confidence, which also affects mental health.

TCM Overview

1. The unbalanced proliferation of Yang energy in the liver.
2. Accumulation of digestive system imbalance.
3. Unbalanced Lung Yin energy.
4. Effects of psychological problems on the digestive system.
5. Imbalance of spleen meridian energy.
6. Mistakes in eating habits, such as eating too much, or starving constantly, eating too quickly, eating at late hours.

Acupoints solution:

PC 6, Nei Guan (内关): Balance heart yang energy, helps to improve psychological problems.

PC 8, Lao Gong (劳宫): Especially to eliminate bad breath.

RN 12, Zhong Wan (中脘): Balance digestive system.

Recommendation:

- Do not eat late.
- Gargle with mint or mild saltwater several times a day.
- If you have diseases of the teeth, mouth, digestive system, get a treatment.
- Have the habit of brushing teeth in the morning and evening.
- Solve the constipation problem.
- Do breathing exercises.
- Make sports a habit.
- Do not be too hungry or too full.
- Good oral hygiene helps prevent bad breath.
- Get advice on mouth care.
- Useful teas and fruits: Ginger tea, two times a day, morning drink on an empty stomach.

> ➤ Lemon-mint tea or clove tea can be drunk a few times a day.
> ➤ Every day eat a handful of jujube fruit (red dates)

Massage technique. For point RN 12, you can put your right hand on the point, open your left hand and deep breath for 10 Minutes.

Headaches

Most people will have headaches in their lives. There are two main types of headache:

Primary headaches, which are not caused by another injury or illness. The reasons can be stress, eyestrain or squinting, poor posture, dehydration, drinking too much alcohol or eating certain foods, lack of sleep, poor posture, skipping a meal.

Secondary headaches which are caused by some underlying health conditions. Such as an illness or a head injury or concussion. Hormones may cause headaches in women. Some headaches can occur as a side effect of medication, such as painkillers. People sometimes get headaches when they're unwell. For example, you may get a headache when you have a cold, sinusitis, flu or an allergic reaction.

TCM diagnosis determines which meridian is connected to the headache, groups headaches according to their reasons, such as cold, hot, windy, or damp, then treats it accordingly.

Acupoints solution:

LI 4, He Gu (合谷): For the whole head and helps reduce nausea.

SI 2, Si Bai (四白): Especially for headaches caused by eye fatigue. You can notice that your eyes see more clearly and you feel better.

SI 3, Hou Xi (后溪): Especially helps for rear head headaches. This is an acupoint that feels sensitive and has a good influence on the cerebral cortex, so it has an extent curative effect.

SP 6, Tai Chong (太冲): It is especially effective against headaches caused by anger and protects from the damage by anger to the liver. It also helps lower blood and head pressure.

BL 60, Kun Lun (昆仑): Especially helps for rear head headaches. It removes toxins that cause headaches.

EX 3, Tai Yang (太阳): Reduce Migraine and another type of headache. It helps the brain and eye fatigue. Reduces blood pressure and reduces anger.

EX 2, Yin Tang (印堂): Calms the spirit, helps for anxiety and stress. It is beneficial for anterior headache and pain caused by sinusitis.

DU 26, Ren Zhong (人中): Balance the whole body, helps calm down.

PC 6, Nei Guan (内关): Helps relieves stress and eliminates stress-related headaches.

DU 20, Bai Hui (百会): Help balance the whole body and reduce the headache.

Recommendation:

- ➤ Always dry your hair after the shower.
- ➤ Avoid cold drinks.

> ➤ Keep track of what you eat and drink for at least a month, try to find something that doesn't make your headache worse.
> ➤ Improve your sleep quality.
> ➤ Avoid excessive stress.
> ➤ Try to meditate.
> ➤ Try to get rid of your anger.
> ➤ Apply the massage as a 10-day cure.
> ➤ See your doctor if you are getting more headaches than usual.

Heat Stroke

Heat stroke is a life-threatening condition in which the body overheats when it can no longer maintain a healthy temperature. The body temperature will rise from about 37°C to above 40.5°C at the movement. The high body temperature in Heat Stroke can lead to organ damage. You can avoid heatstroke by taking precautions in very hot weather. Heatstroke caused by prolonged exposure to heat. You can get heatstroke inside or outside.

When it happens, we need to apply immediate first aid to lower the body temperature as quickly as possible.

Acupoints Solution

DU 26, Ren Zhong (人中): Emergency aid point.

EX 3, Tai Yang (太阳): Preserves brain function, reduces headache.

EX 2, Yin Tang (印堂): Helps to revive.

LU 11, Shao Shang (少商): Restores fitness and consciousness.

LI 4, He Gu (合谷): Relieves nausea and headache.

PC 6, Nei Guan (内关): Relieves chest distress and restlessness.

SP 6, Tai Chong (太冲): Relieves dizziness and dissipates heat from the body.

KI 1, Yong Quan (涌泉): Emergency point and relieves fatigue.

Note: While applying pressure on these points, do not forget to reduce body temperature, remove water loss, and seek immediate medical attention.

Hiccups

You will probably have had hiccups. They can be annoying but are not usually serious and typically go away after a while. If hiccups go on for longer than two days, they are considered to be long-lasting hiccups, which can interfere with eating and sleeping. TCM theory believes hiccups are caused by abnormally raised energy in the digestive system.

Hiccups occur when your diaphragm suddenly and involuntarily contracts or tightens, causing a sharp intake of breath. When this happens, your vocal cords will quickly close, which produces the 'hiccup' sound.

Hiccups may start and stop with no obvious reason. However, some things increase your chances of having hiccups including: overeating, or eating too quickly, spicy foods, hot or fizzy food or drinks, alcohol, smoking, stress, fear or excitement.

In rare cases, hiccups that last for days or weeks. Some underlying conditions, or some medications may cause it. They are: gastro-esophageal reflux (GERD) or heartburn, pneumonia or asthma, brain injury (such as from trauma, a stroke or a tumour), central nervous system disorders, such as multiple sclerosis and stroke metabolic disorders, such as diabetes. some medications.

Long-lasting hiccups can cause discomfort and pain, disrupt sleeping and eating, and may cause anxiety or depression. So, it's very important to learn how to stop hiccups.

TCM overview

Stomach energy stagnation, reverse, having cold energy in the stomach. Acupoints Solutions

LU 11, Shao Shang (少商): Very effective for sudden onset hiccups. Pressed on the point with two middle fingers to take a deep breath, we hold the breath as long as it can and keep pressing. Apply one or two times.

PC 6, Nei Guan (内关): Gives inner peace, regular the nervous system.

RN 12, Zhong Wan (中脘): Helps to reduce gastroesophageal reflux (GERD) or heartburn symptoms.

Recommendation

Avoid food and drink that are too cold or too hot.

If your hiccups last longer than two days, see your doctor. If an underlying condition is causing your hiccups, treating it may help.

If you have a lengthy period of hiccups, and your treatment didn't give a result, do your massage as a 10-15-day cure. Acupuncture treatments can help stop long-lasting hiccups.

Hypertension

TCM Overview

The TCM belief is that high blood pressure, caused by the liver and meridian, heart and meridian imbalance. The reason is anger, excessive stress, malnutrition, drinking, smoking and irregular lifestyle that cause excessive yang energy in the liver. The reason for the blockage of the heart meridian energy is inactivity and restlessness, and a lack of inner peace. Nutritional problems / poor nutrition, for example, too much fat, not enough vegetables, cause the edema to accumulate and affect blood pressure.

Acupoints Solution

EX 21, Er Jian (耳尖): Positive effect on blood pressure.

DU 20, Bai Hui (百会): It maintains the balance of the whole body and reduces the excess energy in the head.

LI 11, Qu Qi (曲池): Reduces excessive heat in the body, reduces pressure.

PC 6, Nei Guan (内关): It reduces the pressure in the heart, protects the heart and gives inner peace.

HT 7, Shen Men (神门): Restores inner peace and relieves excessive stress.

SP 6, San Yin Jiao (三阴交): Reduces edema, detoxifies.

LI 3, Tai Chong (太冲): It provides inner peace by reducing the anger and ensures the liver to function regularly.

Gao Xue Ya Dian (高血压点): It directly affects blood pressure to go back to regular.

DU 26, Ren Zhong (人中): It can be used when you are not yet able to get medical help. This is an emergency acupoint.

Recommendations

> ➤ Get to bed early, and get up early, pay attention to the biological clock.

- ➤ Take care of your diet.
- ➤ Have regular check-ups, measure blood pressure regularly.
- ➤ Do regular walking and sports.
- ➤ Listen to music that will bring peace.
- ➤ Stay away from things that will ruin your inner peace.
- ➤ Get rid of constipation.
- ➤ Watch your weight.
- ➤ Avoid smoking and alcohol.
- ➤ Do meditation.
- ➤ When you do things for your health, please do it regularly.
- ➤ Learn to control your anger.

Caution: Do not stop using the medicine you are using

Hypotension (Low blood pressure)

As the heart pumps blood around the body, the pressure with which it pushes against the walls of blood vessels changes. When the heart is squeezing blood into the arteries, the pressure is high. When the heart is relaxed, the pressure is lower. For some people, low blood pressure is a sign of good health. These are people who are very fit and who have a slow pulse. But for others, low blood pressure is a problem.

The symptoms of low blood pressure may include: Lightheadedness, dizziness, weakness, blurred vision, pale, clammy skin, fatigue, sometimes fainting.

People can have low blood pressure if they: are overheated, have too little blood circulating from donating blood or from being dehydrated, have drugs or alcohol in the body system, are in severe pain, or have nutritional deficiencies.

TCM overview

Yang energy deficiency, Insufficient cardiac drive, spleen, and kidney energy deficiency.

Acupoints Solution

KI 1, Yong Quan (涌泉): Helps increase energy level.

BL 60, Kun Lun (昆仑): Balances blood pressure.

DU 26, Ren Zhong (人中): The first aid point regulates fallen blood pressure.

DU 20, Bai Hui (百会): Especially useful for light-headedness, dizziness.

DU 25, Su Liao (素寥): Maintains a heart rhythm., regulates fallen blood pressure.

RN 17, Dan Zhong (膻中): Reduce the pressure behind the sternum and give a sense of tranquillity.

Recommendation:

- ➢ Avoiding dehydration, hot showers, or standing up too quickly.
- ➢ Try to do sport regularly or learn qigong exercises and do it.

However, if you experience continuing symptoms of low blood pressure, you should see a doctor. If there is an underlying cause for your low blood pressure, and it is giving you problems, you may need treatment for that underlying cause.

Leg cramps

TCM Overview

According to TCM, the Spleen controls muscles and extremities, Liver controls tendons, and Kidney controls bone. If these organs' energy is weak, there are muscle, bone and tendon problems in the body. Such as cold and dampness, stagnation of meridians or other stimuli, resulting in lower extremity meridian energy and blood, maybe cramps on legs.

So, principle for treatment is, open the meridians, remove the blockage, get rid of the cold and dampness, balance spleen, liver and kidney meridians energy.

Acupoints Solution

BL 40, Wei Zhong (委中): Detoxification, nourish muscles of legs.

BL 57, Cheng Shan (承山): Relieve muscle excitement, nourish muscles of legs, Improves local blood circulation.

KI 1, Yong Quan (涌泉): Balance kidney meridians energy.

SP 6, Tai Chong (太冲): Balance liver meridians energy.

Recommendations

- ➤ Stay active but do proper warm-ups and cool-downs before and after exercise.
- ➤ Avoid overtraining and build in plenty of rest for proper muscle recovery as a preventative measure.
- ➤ Stay hydrated. Drink enough water every day based on your body size. This helps prevent muscle problems caused by heat exhaustion, intense thirst or heavy sweating.
- ➤ Weight loss if you are carrying excess weight
- ➤ When the weather is cold, pay attention to the cold and warmth of the lower limbs.

> ➤ Older people should get out in the sun.
> ➤ Try to relax.

Loss of appetite (anorexia)

Appetite is the normal need of the body for food. This need manifests by hunger. With the digestion of food in a healthy person, glucose in the blood rises and a feeling of fullness occurs. But sometimes, the appetite may temporarily disappear. Likely causes are stress and excessive fatigue, unhealthy habits (alcohol, smoking), not eating regularly, eating cold food constantly, disturbed sleep patterns, some medications and diseases.

TCM Overview

Chinese medicine believes that if the external factors of the body have destroyed the internal factors, and caused the imbalance in the body, the spleen and stomach are not coordinated, resulting in insufficient energy and decreased appetite.

Acupoints solution:

ST 25, Tian Shu (天枢): Regulates the flow of energy in the abdomen.

DU 20, Bai Hui (百会): Helps balance the whole-body energy.

EX 28, Si Feng (四缝): Stimulate appetite, especially for babies and children.

ST 36, Zu San Li (足三里): Strengthens and harmonises the Spleen and Stomach, clears food stagnation, makes contracting Qi descend, enhances immune function.

RN 12, Zhong Wan (中脘): Balance digestive system.

RN 8, Shen Que (神阙): It awakens exhausted energy again.

Recommendation:

➤ Avoid Stress;
➤ Do Sports;
➤ Do not drink much water before eating;
➤ Don't start the day without breakfast;
➤ Do not wait for meals to eat, try to eat immediately when you feel hungry.

Use some spices to raise your appetite: Hot red pepper, Coriander, Ginger, Anise, Cumin.

Loss of libido (reduced sex drive)

Loss of libido is a common problem that affects many men and women at some point in their life. Common causes of low libido are: Ejaculation problems, erectile dysfunction, vaginal dryness, painful sex, inability to orgasm, involuntary tightening of the vagina (vaginismus), stress, anxiety, and exhaustion. A low sex drive can also be a side effect of antidepressants. Falling levels of sex hormones (testosterone) in men age-related health problems. Falling levels of sex hormones (estrogen and testosterone) just before, during and after the menopause in women. Pregnancy, giving birth and breastfeeding, loss of interest in sex is common during pregnancy, after giving birth and while breastfeeding. It is often linked to relationship issues, stress or tiredness, but can be a sign of an underlying medical problem, such as reduced hormone levels.

TCM Overview

In TCM, the belief is that your life energy is not strong enough, and that kidney and liver energy are unbalanced.

Acupoints Solution

DU 3, Yao Yang Guan (腰阳关): Increases your life energy.

RN 4, Guan Yuan (关元): Increases life energy, balances genitalia energy.

SP 6, San Yin Jiao (三阴交): Balances spleen, kidney and liver meridians, reduces stress, makes you feel vigorous.

KI 1, Yong Quan (涌泉): Regulate kidney meridian's energy, let you feel energetics.

Recommendations:

Do the horse stance exercise-sometimes called horse-riding stance.

This is a Chinese martial arts stance. Be calm, breathe naturally, deep and steady, to exercise the chest, kidney and to indent the abdominal muscles and create muscle tension in the legs.

1. Stand with feet apart and the legs wide the distance between the two feet is the length of the two soles of the feet, then squat, the toes are parallel forward. Bend the knees forwards, the knees don't extend beyond the toes, and the thighs are parallel to the ground.
2. Adduct the thighs as though you are gripping a horse between your legs.
3. Keep the back and head in a vertical line.

Note: Exercise at least once a day, and the cumulative time for each exercise can start from five minutes and rise to 30 minutes. Use the above work as a 10-14 days cure.

Menopause

Menopause is the time that marks the end of your menstrual cycles. Menopause can happen in your 40s or 50s. It is a natural biological process, but the physical symptoms, such as hot flushes, and emotional symptoms may disrupt your sleep, lower your energy or affect emotional health.

Women in menopause might experience these signs and symptoms: Irregular periods, vaginal dryness, hot flushes, chills, night sweats, sleep problems, mood changes, weight gain and slowed metabolism, thinning hair and dry skin, loss of breast fullness. Skipping periods during perimenopause is common and expected. Often, menstrual periods will skip a month and return, or skip several months and then start monthly cycles again for a few months. Periods also happen on shorter cycles, so they are closer together. Despite irregular periods, pregnancy is possible. If you've skipped a period but aren't sure you've started the menopausal transition, consider a pregnancy test.

TCM Overview

Chinese medicine believes menopause is a situation called 'Before and after menopause syndrome'. That is a pathological change in physiological conditions. Kidney energy deficiency is the basis, other reasons are yin and yang energy disorders. Treatment aimed at strengthening the organ's harmony, balances the kidney, liver, heart, and spleen meridian's energy. Maintaining the balance of the body, find a solution for the complaint, bringing inner peace.

Acupoints Solution

DU 20, Bai Hui (百会): Helps you control yourself, gives you peace of mind, improves concentration.

PC 6, Nei Guan (内关): Gives inner peace, regular the nervous system.

Li 11, Qu Qi (曲池): Reduce hot flush, sweating and skin dryness.

SP 10, Xue Hai (血海): Keeps the blood structure in balance, cooling the body.

SP 6, San Yin Jiao (三阴交): It removes toxins and cools the body. Increases body resistance. Help keep sleep quality high. Reduces edema.

DU 4, Ming Men (命门): Strengthens the energy of life, gives vitality, brings happiness.

Recommendations:

 ➢ Get information that menopause is a normal physiological process.
 ➢ Don't panic, try to do things that make you happy.
 ➢ Try to get family support, a healthy family relationship will give you peace of mind.
 ➢ Find activities you love to engage in.
 ➢ Take a walk, watch your weight, avoid gaining weight.
 ➢ Avoid excessive tea and coffee.
 ➢ Don't watch horror and hyper-emotional movies.
 ➢ Listen to relaxing music, meet and chat with friends.
 ➢ Go outside and experience the beauty of nature.
 ➢ Do not move away from your sexual life.
 ➢ Ask your doctor about proper nutrition.
 ➢ Pay more attention to teeth, skin and body cleaning, take care of yourself.
 ➢ Take time for yourself and value yourself.
 ➢ Do not neglect to have a routine check-up.
 ➢ Measure your blood pressure regularly.

- ➤ Wear cotton and be healthy.
- ➤ Do breathing exercises.
- ➤ Do meditation every day

Painful periods (Dysmenorrhea)

Many women will experience pain during their period. It is very common in young women. Menstruation causes period pains, and most commonly causes pain in the lower abdominal area. Sometimes this pain spreads towards the back and thigh areas.

The pain may feel like sharp twinges or constant, dull pain. And the discomfort and aches, there are also several other symptoms that you may experience during your period, such as headache, tiredness, nausea, dizziness, diarrhea, feeling faint.

TCM Overview

Low energy in blood circulation, unbalanced operation or blockage of spleen, liver, kidney meridians. They make the solution from these places.

Acupoints Solution

ST 36, Zu San Li (足三里): Helps increase energy.

SP 1, Yin Bai (隐白): Regulates blood circulation.

SP 6, San Yin Jiao (三阴交): Balances spleen, Kidney and Liver meridians, dissolves congestion, reduces stress.

ST 25, Tian Shu (天枢): Regulates the flow of energy in the abdomen.

SP 10, Xue Hai (血海): Invigorates and moves the Blood, regulates menstruation.

KI 1, Yong Quan (涌泉): Regulate kidney meridian's energy, let you feel good.

DU 20, Bai Hui (百会): Reduces and relieves headaches and stress.

Recommendations:

➤ Breathing exercise: Deep diaphragm breathing exercise performed every day for 5-10 minutes.
➤ We should always keep the abdomen and Waist warm.
➤ Do not drink cold drinks from the refrigerator during menstruation.
➤ Use massage technique or moxa.

Note

Use the above as a 7- 10 days treatment. Do not massage your abdomen during menstruation

Palpitations

Often, our hearts develop their own rhythm and we are not aware of it. Palpitations can range from being aware of your heart's activity to the sensation of it beating faster and harder than usual. It can sometimes feel like your heart is missing beats.

Causes of palpitations include stress, emotional changes, anxious, including panic attacks. This is due to a rise in adrenaline levels, which can cause your heart to beat faster. Exercise, strenuous activity, drinks or foods containing caffeine, alcohol, some medicines, low blood sugar, anaemia, sudden low blood pressure. It is an unpleasant sensation, bringing fear, excitement, or anxiety, building itself up.

TCM Overview

TCM believes that sudden emotional changes, long-term illness, irregular nutrition and life, disturbance of sleep patterns are reasons for palpitations. The treatment is to gain inner peace, by getting used to living with a regular routine and getting rid of fear.

Acupoints Solution

DU 25, Su Liao (素髎): Help corrects palpitations. Note: This point is suitable for adults, not for children.

PC 6, Nei Guan (内关): Gives inner peace, nourishes the heart, cleanses fear. Especially help regulation of cardiovascular activity.

HT 7, Shen Men (神门): Improves sleep quality, adjusts the autonomic nervous system (ANS), calms your mind and gives inner peace.

DU 20, Bai Hui (百会): It is useful to get rid of fear and to control the body.

Note: These points work well for the relief of palpitations. They point will strengthen its positive effect of medication. If you are not taking the medication, it will bring you peace of mind in a short time. Or they will help you until you see your doctor. If you are very excited, you can also use it to soothe excitement, to gain a feeling of inner peace and to avoid palpitations.

Recommendation:

➢ Exercise regularly
➢ Avoid excessive alcohol use
➢ Keep hydrated, drink enough water
➢ Practice meditation and deep breathing.

See your doctor if the palpitations are more than a couple of seconds, get worse, if you have heart problems or severe shortness of breath, chest pain or dizziness.

Quit smoking

The adverse symptoms and diseases caused by smoking vary from distressing to fatal. Too numerous to mention here. Damage and disruption occur to every organ, tissue and physiological system, including mental and emotional health.

Acupoints Solution

LU 7, Lie Que (列缺): It is an effective experience acupoint in smoking cessation.

Li 11, Qu Qi (曲池): Detox acupoint, reduces the harm of smoking.

DU 20, Bai Hui (百会): Improves self-control ability, helps to break smoking.

HT 7, Shen Men (神门): Reduces the desire for cigarettes, reduces stress and has a sedative effect.

Note:

Touching the Lie Que acupoint when you want to smoke will reduce or eliminate your desire to smoke. In the meantime, the practice of breathing exercises will also help you.

If you are receiving treatment for smoking cessation, these acupoints will support your treatment.

Reducing Appetite (To Aid Healthy Weight Loss)

All of us hope to maintain our normal weight. Who doesn't want to have a healthy and beautiful appearance, strong self-confidence feeling, a light body that allows us to move comfortably, less risk of illness, and a physique that positively affects our mental health?

Some people's weight problem depends on the disease. Even so, you can still use these acupoints and get the benefit. It can help support your doctor and treatment to cure your current illness.

Acupoints Solution

ST 4, Di Cang (地仓): Gives a feeling of satiety and helps to control hunger.

RN24, Cheng Jian (承浆): Helps to secrete saliva and facilitates digestion.

HT 7, Shen Men (神门): Reduces stress and reduces aggression towards food.

RN 12, Zhong Wan (中脘): Gives a feeling of feeling full and keeps the digestive system working balance.

GB 31, Feng Shi (风市): Has a positive effect on fat metabolism.

Recommendation:

➤ Don't eat late.
➤ Consume easy to digest food.
➤ Look after your own nutrition.
➤ Trust yourself.
➤ Don't try to lose weight quickly.
➤ Eat less and slowly.
➤ Serve your food to your plate only once.
➤ Exercise regularly.
➤ Drink enough water, make sure your urine colour is light.

➢ Get a meridian massage for a balanced system and metabolism.

➢ You are not losing anything; you are gaining energy and freedom.

Sleep problems

TCM Overview

1. Emotional problems make liver energy stagnate, causing uneasy feelings, and affect sleep. 2. The diet is not adjusted, the food is stagnant, and the stomach is out of balance, affecting sleep.

2. A long illness makes the whole-body energy insufficient, special is heart energy deficient, the reason is anxiety, affects sleep.

3. Feelings of guilt and fear disturbing inner peace, affect sleep.

Therefore, the principle of treatment is to regulate the yin and yang energy disorders of the heart, liver, gallbladder, spleen, stomach, and kidney meridians.

Acupoints Solution

HT 7, Shen Men (神门): It rests the soul and opens the closed soul door. Improves sleep quality.

SP 6, San Yin Jiao (三阴交): Improves sleep quality with detox effect PC 6, Nei Guan (内关): Improves sleep quality by providing inner peace.

DU 20, Bai Hui (百会): It teaches us to control ourselves, removes insomnia-causing thoughts.

SP 6, Tai Chong (太冲): Reduces anger, removes toxins that cause insomnia.

Recommendations

➤ Balance between overwork and rest, take time for yourself, maintain the right balance between work and daily life.

➤ Respect your biological clock.

➤ Go to sleep early and get up early.

➤ Don't eat late.

➤ Avoid having an empty life.

➤ Be sincere to yourself and your surroundings.

➤ Avoid the factors that negatively affect your sleep.

➤ Listen to your favourite relaxing.

➤ Don't smoke.

➤ Stay away from things that will disturb your conscience.

➤ Do not ignore your problem, share it or consult a doctor.

➤ Sports, exercise.

Stiff Neck

Neck pain is a common condition that will affect most people in their lives. Many things can cause neck pain. The pain often spreads from the neck towards the shoulders or upper back, sometimes causing headaches.

Common causes of neck pain include: poor posture, sleeping in an awkward position, tension, injury such as a muscle strain, leaving hair wet, prolonged use of a desktop or laptop computer, arthritis, wear and tear in the bones of the neck.

TCM Overview

Bladder, Kidney, Liver meridians energy blocked. Chronic injury. Poor posture. Wind and Cold factors on the neck muscles.

Acupoints Solution:

LI 4, He Gu (合谷): Especially used when the headache is added with neck pain.

Li 11, Qu Qi (曲池): Counteract inflammation, regulates blood circulation for the area.

SI 3, Hou Xi (后溪): Especially helps for rear head headaches. This is an acupoint that feels sensitive and has a good influence on the cerebral cortex and neck.

SI 11, Tian Zong (天宗): When you have pain in the scapular region.

Lao Zhen Xue (落枕穴): It is a special point for neck pain.

Ashi Points: Warm the sorest spot or area using the palm of your hand.

Recommendation:

➢ Protect the neck from wind.
➢ Always dry your hair.
➢ Take care of your posture.
➢ Exercise and massage should be done regularly.
➢ Use suitable pillows.
➢ Avoid excessive stress.
➢ Practice breathing and meditate.
➢ Do not carry heavy objects.
➢ Avoid extreme sports.

You need to see your doctor if:

1. The pain is getting worse
2. The pain doesn't ease up in a week

3. You have numbness, tingling or pins, and needles in your arms or legs
4. You have difficulties with your bladder or bowel;
5. You have a fever and neck pain.

Stress

Everyone knows about the damage done to people by excessive stress. In fact, stress is a normal part of human nature. It is an energy that inspires us to do something, gives us the desire to learn and succeed, and gives us the strength to overcome fear. A small amount of stress, such as meeting a challenge or deadline can be helpful. It can lead to increased alertness, energy and productivity. A complete lack of stress can lead to reduced motivation and performance.

Chinese medicine believes that excessive pressure causes insufficient functioning of life energy and that heart energy is lacking. When our heart is not taken care of, our soul cannot be nourished well. That the soul cannot be fed well creates congestion in energy. When your soul does not feed well, the body energy may clog. Lack of energy causes the imbalance of other organs. Unbalanced and low levels of energy produced affect the spleen, lungs, liver, kidneys and even the brain. Therefore, fatigue, restlessness, disturbance of sleep patterns, a feeling of weight in the head, breathing failure, palpitations, fatigue, reluctance, and many other complaints are caused by stress. That's why people who seem young and healthy are feeling old. The treatment is to maintain the balance of the body Yin and Yang, support the heart and spleen, strengthen kidney energy, detox, and provide peace of mind.

There are many ways to manage stress, including identifying your triggers, acupuncture, relaxation techniques, lifestyle changes and seeking support from others. If you are feeling overwhelmed by stress and unable to cope, seek advice from a counsellor or health professional.

Acupoints Solution

DU 20, Bai Hui (百会): It allows self-control, calms, prevents forgetfulness and helps concentration.

PC 6, Nei Guan (内关): Creates a peaceful feeling, stops palpitations.

HT 7, Shen Men (神门): It calms the soul.

SP 6, San Yin Jiao (三阴交): Creates vitality, relieves tiredness, reduces stress and creates a feeling of happiness.

SP 6, Tai Chong (太冲): It takes away anger, makes a feeling of being purified and cleansed. Relieves pressure. Increases patience.

Recommendations:

➢ Continue the above points massage for 10 days.
➢ Drink plenty of water.

Tinnitus

Ringing or other strange noises in your ears. It is very annoying. Tinnitus can come and go, or you might experience it continuously. It can come from hearing loss, ear wax, exposure to loud noises, ear infections, some diseases, and medicines. Stress, anxiety, and caffeine can make it worse.

TCM Overview

They consider that it relates this to the insufficiency of Kidney Meridian's energy. Because the kidney opens in the ear, it reflects the energy from the ear. If it is not caused by another disease, usually the method used in tinnitus is to raise kidney meridians energy.

Acupoints Solution:

SI 19, Ting Gong (听宫): Balances ear function.

SJ 3, Zhong Zhu (中渚): Balances ear function and it is a special point for treating tinnitus.

KI 1, Yong Quan (涌泉): Perfect for raising kidney and whole-body energy.

Recommendations:

Breathing exercise: Place hands on both ears, take a deep breath with a focus on Umbilical. Tighten your belly when breathing in, lower it when breathing out. Do this process between 5 and 10 minutes each day. If your body or ear warms up during this exercise, you've done it.

Note

You need to do this for 10 days. You can interrupt. After 10 days, repeat.

Toothache

Many people know that acupuncture is a very effective method of a general toothache. It is a safe, inexpensive and easy.

Toothache can start suddenly. It can cause pain and discomfort that ranges from mild to very severe. The pain may affect not only your tooth but also your head, ear, and jaw. The pain may be constant, throbbing, or it may come and go.

If you have a toothache, it could be caused by:

1. Tooth decay
2. A cracked tooth
3. A loose filling or a broken filling
4. Inflammation of the pulp inside your tooth
5. Receding gums
6. An abscess
7. Sinus infection

TCM Overview

Need to balance patients' stomach and kidney meridian.

Acupoints Solution:

LI 4, He Gu (合谷): Relieves pain.

KI 3, Tai Xi (太溪): Benefits of reducing inflammation and swelling, especially good for the relief of toothache.

SP 1, Yin Bai (隐白): Help stop bleeding gums.

DU 26, Ren Zhong (人中): Good for upper toothache.

EX 21, Er Jian (耳尖): Experience point for toothache.

SP 6, San Yin Jiao (三阴交): Anti-inflammatory, balance kidney meridians, strengthens the immune system.

Recommendations

- ➤ Have regular dental care.
- ➤ Make sure you keep your teeth and mouth clean, rinse your mouth after every meal.
- ➤ Brush your teeth twice a day, use a soft toothbrush.
- ➤ Avoid drinks that are too hot or too cold.

- Lie with your head propped up on a pillow, as lying flat can sometimes make dental pain feel worse.
- Saltwater wash 2-3 times per day. Mix one teaspoon of salt into a cup of warm water, then take a mouthful of the liquid and hold it in your mouth so it covers your affected tooth for two minutes, then spit it out. Do not swallow it.
- Saltwater should not for children because they may accidentally swallow it.
- Avoid wind.

Vomiting

Vomiting can happen for many reasons. A viral infection, food poisoning, illness or pregnancy can all cause vomiting. Vomiting in adults is usually not a sign of anything serious and usually improves within 48 hours (two days), but it is an annoying situation. It can be a sign of something more serious.

TCM overview

TCM said the ingestion of harmful substances from outside, a weakening and unbalanced energy of spleen and stomach function is the reason for vomiting. When the body can't accept something for body systems, it will push out the things that have bad energy. So, the treatment principles are evil dispelling and letting the energy flow in the right way.

Acupoints Solution

PC 6, Nei Guan (内关): Regular stomach energy.

ST 36, Zu San Li (足三里): Provides to balance of digestive system function.

RN 12, Zhong Wan (中脘): It allows the stomach energy to go in the right direction.

LI 4, He Gu (合谷): Keeps the path open of the nutrients that should go.

Recommendation:

People who frequently vomit should pay attention to their food. Should avoid food that is too greasy and difficult to digest. Should not eat much. Avoid cold, bitter and spicy foods. Food should be consumed fresh.

See your doctor if:

1. The vomiting lasts for over 24 hours;
2. You have had bouts of nausea and vomiting over the last month;
3. You are losing a lot of weight;
4. You think it dehydrated you;
5. Have a fever or projectile vomiting.

Note: Pregnant ladies should not use the acupoints.

Wrist pain

The wrist joint plays a role in basic movements, from texting to writing. It contains many muscles and tendons at the joint of the bones that make up the arm. Elbow pain prevents the person from performing the simplest daily movements and reduces the quality of life.

Recurring wrist pain is often due to conditions, such as repetitive stress injuries and inflammation of the joints. Causes can be carpal tunnel syndrome, osteoarthritis, rheumatoid arthritis, repetitive motion syndrome, tendonitis, bursitis, or sprain.

TCM Overview

It is a principle in TCM that if there is a blockage in energy, there will be pain.

Acupoints solution:

PC 6, Nei Guan (内关): Relieves wrist pain. Because the median nerve lies directly beneath this point, so you need to avoid hard pressure.

SJ 5, Wai Guan (外关): Relieves wrist pain, protects deformation.

LI 11, Qu Qi (曲池): Counteract inflammation, regulates blood circulation for the area.

Recommendation:

- ➢ Exercise regularly; If you have the symptoms as below, please see a doctor:
- ➢ Pain is interfering with everyday activities.
- ➢ Numbness or tingling is becoming worse, and there is little or no feeling in the fingers or hand.
- ➢ Simple hand movements are no longer possible.
- ➢ Weakness makes holding things difficult.

My Top 10 Acupoints

You will have noticed that some points are used for different and unrelated ailments. One reason is that the same action, for example moving sluggish Qi, can treat many symptoms.

Another is that the point has a beneficial effect on general health, mood, and emotions.

Here are 10 points I like to use on my patients and myself on a regular basis.

DU 20, Bai Hui (百会): It allows me to control myself, calms me down, prevents my forgetfulness and helps my concentration.

EX 3, Tai Yang (太阳): Rests my brain, takes away my eye fatigue.

ST 2, Si Bai (四白): Reduces eye fatigue, brightens the eye, makes me see more clearly.

PC 6, Nei Guan (内关): Makes me feel peaceful, in safety, helps stop my palpitations.

HT 3, Shao Hai (少海): Helps my fears go away.

RN 17, Dan Zhong (膻中): Gives me a feeling of happiness, reduces sadness.

Li 11, Qu Qi (曲池): Nourishes the skin, warms me when I'm cold and cools me down when I am feeling

hot.

RN 4, Guan Yuan (关元): Makes me feel energetic.

SP 6, San Yin Jiao (三阴交): Makes me feel healthy, gives me vitality, relieves my tiredness, reduces my

stress and gives me a feeling of happiness.

SP 6, Tai Chong (太冲): Helps to detox, relieves my anger, keep my liver healthy. It makes me feel purified and cleansed, relieves the physical feeling of pressure, and makes me more patient.

I keep them in my pocket like the saviour medicine. They give me peace, happiness, and vitality in daily life, reassuring me on the journey. They help me calm down in case of an emergency. They help to detox, relieve my anger, and keep my liver healthy.

A reminder

Let's not forget that we only use them to improve our quality of life. You shouldn't neglect modern medicine. If needed, consult your doctor, because you may need medical treatment. When Western Medicine and Traditional Medicine become friends, supporting each other, it is possible to gain even more health and a long healthy life.

CHAPTER 6
Ra Qi Therapy

Ra-Qi is a therapy I have been developing since 2004. It can be described as the balancing of body systems. I would like to share what I have learned in the past years, as well as my ideas of how beneficial the process could be for patients, the health care system and the population.

For many years, in Turkey, I worked almost solely with acupuncture. Although it is very good for certain types of disorders, some of my patients would have questions and problems that acupuncture couldn't address. For example, people with a low pain threshold. Also, some people change their minds as soon as they hear it involves needles, and some of them stop treatment after only a couple of days.

In light of this, I remembered Hippocrates philosophy *'Primum non nocere'*, first do no harm. I believe this is the first thing a doctor should do when treating the patient. I came up with an idea, with minimal pain on the part of the patient and no use of needles.

As I was thinking of developing a new therapy method, a patient came along with her daughter. The mother said: "My girl will not use needles under any circumstances and because of complications she's not able to take any medication either. She's underperforming at school because of her migraine, which makes her sad. I came to you hoping you could treat my daughter without any needles or medication, through massage".

Until then I used to add in a little massage where necessary but had never used it as a primary tool. I used pressure on the acupuncture points as massage therapy. After the first session, the patient was feeling considerably better. After seven sessions, we were both so happy about the result.

Since then, I started incorporating more acupressure and massaging, and less use of needles. I was amazed at the results. I was getting better responses from other patients with fewer sessions. Sometimes the sessions comprised massage only. Meanwhile, society was becoming more aware about healing touch, so I decided to call upon my Qi Gong training and incorporated it into my sessions. The results were ever improving with lots of positive feedback. Even healthy people came to feel more energetic and alive.

Over the years I have been able to combine several methods and develop a fixed progression which I now call **Ra-Chi Therapy**. It is a combination of acupressure, massage, Qi Gong and Reiki. I have created a treatment regime where the beneficial effects are much stronger than the sum of its parts.

How Ra Qi therapy Works

At the initial consultation, I check the patients' chakras to see where they might have a problem. In the early stages, I used a pendulum. In healthy people and healthy chakras, the pendulum turns slightly clockwise, in ill or psychologically unstable people, the pendulum has unpredictable motion. For example, for yin type symptoms, the pendulum doesn't move at all. Where for yang type symptoms, the pendulum shakes or rotates clockwise. In this way I can predict patients with their chakra's points or the corresponding organs. Thus, I am able to determine where or what kind of disorder a patient has. Such a method of diagnosing helps me to gain the patient's trust and successfully completes the first step in recovery.

The second step is the therapy process. I have started using technics massage on channels, 5 of which are located on the back. I also made it a priority to use Traditional Chinese meridians and the important acupoints on them. As we mentioned earlier, some of these acupoints represent our organs and even emotions. Therefore, when I find a painful or sense of changed acupoint during the massage, I can tell the patient the problems a related organ might have. In such cases, my patients ask how I know about their complaints. The success of the treatment is improved yet again.

The third step is followed by a focused massage on the painful acupoints, which I will refer to as 'messenger' acupoints from here on. Since the points I find relate to specific problems in the patient's body, I give them advice on what they can do at home. From the information gathered by messenger points, I tell the patients which organ is sensitive for them, and what they can do to improve them, such as massage the points at home or exercise and breathing exercises.

The fourth step involves adjusting the energy in certain parts of the body, including the chakras. Some patients enjoy this part so much and say it's the 'Finale'.

A typical session as described takes between 30-50 minutes. As a result, I have developed a unique, non-invasive therapy that can produce visible results, making my patients happy and healthy quickly.

Ra Qi is easy to learn and use. It helps people understand that the body, like a machine, needs maintenance and repairing now and then. Apart from its health benefits, Ra Qi helps people attain a state of emotional wellbeing, develop their potential, motivate them to a healthy lifestyle, improve inter-personal relationships, and develop a true sense of happiness.

The advantages of Ra Qi Therapy are that it can treat patients successfully without any side-effects and, being non-invasive, is a useful tool in people with a fear of needles and pain. In some cases, it can help a course of treatment by decreasing the need to use pills or medication. It is an excellent practice to prevent illness.

Ra Qi therapy is an excellent way to detoxify, and is beneficial in preparing patients for surgery, as well as post-operative recovery.

Patients benefit from the doctor's touch. They need attention not only on bodily functions but also on an emotional and mental level. Along with the treatment they need support, recommendations, and an overall solution.

I believe Ra Qi therapy will go a long way to creating a healthy, and health-motivated, society.

Case Study

This 35-year-old owner of a tourism company had a great love for her work and family. She had experienced some serious problems 3-4 months before she came to me. She realised that she had become a different person, so she came to me.

She didn't want to go to work, didn't want to wake up, and when she forced herself to go to work, even had fights with the employees. Her performance at work was constantly dropping. She also started having marital problems. She couldn't stand her husband and didn't even want to see him. She was even neglecting her 5 years old son. As the problems grew, she eventually came to the stage where she didn't go to work and had serious fights with her husband. She was aware she was causing the problems and was regretful of doing so.

She didn't want to see a doctor for two reasons. First, she was not willing to use prescribed pharmaceutical medicine. Also, the person who advised her to go to the doctor was her husband. After understanding how serious her problem was, she started searching for doctors that could work without medication. She came to me with many questions in her head.

The first thing she said was "I want to get a single treatment just to try, but I absolutely don't want any needles". She was wondering what I would do to her body and if she would ever feel like the previous years when she was healthy and happy. I replied "If we don't use our body properly, it is like a field covered with weeds. Unbalanced energy pollution prohibits our body from utilising the oxygen and the nutrients correctly. It would look like barren sand without water and life. Now we will pull the weeds out of your body field, then let the water, oxygen, and the nutrients flow freely".

During the first session, she started feeling the weight being taken off from her shoulders bit by bit. After therapy, she suddenly felt lighter. She even realised her eyes were seeing more clearly. She decided to come to more sessions because she felt so good. After 7 sessions once a week, she was back to her former self - a wonderful mother, a suitable wife, and a successful young boss again.

She said, "I am emotionally newborn again!".

CHAPTER 7

Principles and Daily Treatment for a Healthy and Happy Life

Morning Routine

To do these little things, you only need to get up 10-15 minutes early from your normal time.

First, open the window to allow air exchange and light to enter, drink a glass of warm water, then gently rub your whole body. This will revitalise your stagnant energy from the night and give you vitality. It will provide the best flow of energy in the meridians.

Best results are achieved by doing it in order. Head-neck-chest-abdomen-back-left arm-right arm-left leg-right leg-feet. Please do not rush this practice.

Then, gentle massage or press these points.

EX 3, Tai Yang (太阳) point at the head,

PC 6, Nei Guan (内关) point at the forearm

KI 1, Yong Quan (涌泉) point on the sole of the foot.

By doing this, you will be more productive, energetic and peaceful during the day.

When you can do this exercise at least five times a week, after maybe just 2 or 3 weeks you will notice that your energy has changed, and you are becoming much more positive.

Let's not forget breakfast. Breakfast is like 'opening the fountain'. It kick-starts the stagnant energy from night and provides daylong energy.

During the Day

Acupoints you can massage when you are at work or working from home:

1. To alleviate boredom: **DU 20, Bai Hui (百会), PC 6, Nei Guan (内关), HT 7, Shen Men (神门)**
2. To remove weight in the head: **EX 3, Tai Yang – (太阳), DU 20, Bai Hui (百会).**
3. To relieve fatigue: **KI 1, Yong Quan (涌泉).**
4. To relieve the feeling of weight in your body: **LI 11, Qu Qi (曲池), SP 6, San Yin Jiao (三阴交)**
5. For eye strain: **EX 3, Tai Yang – (太阳), ST 2, Si Bai (四白).**
6. To eliminate smoking: **LU 7, Lie Que (列缺), LI 11, Qu Qi (曲池).**

Note: You can learn how to apply these in Chapter 4. Choose the acupoints that suit you, and use them as needed. If you take a 3-minute '"acupoints break', these points will help you overcome distress and tiredness.

As the Day Ends

We need to do something to relieve the tiredness of the day and invest in the next day. All you need to do is to spend 10-20 minutes and respect your own value. You can even do these while watching TV.

1. For a deep and peaceful sleep: **PC 6, Nei Guan** (内关), **HT 7, Shen Men** (神门).
2. To rest the brain: **DU 20, Bai Hui** (百会), **EX 3, Tai Yang** (太阳).
3. To relieve anger: **LR 3, Tai Chong** (太冲).
4. To relieve the tiredness of the day and to get the day more fit: **KI 1, Yong Quan** (涌泉).

If you hold your warmed palm at your **Yong Quan (KI 1)** point for a minute or two, you will restore your energy and wake up energetic the next day. More productive, healthy, happy days are waiting for you.

Boosting Energy, Being More Dynamic

If you are feeling tired all the time and lacking motivation, these four points can give you energy, hope and willpower.

DU 20, Bai Hui (百会)

EX 3, Tai Yang (太阳)

KI 1, Yong Quan (涌泉)

ST 36, Zu San Li (足三里)

Acupoints for complete detoxification to cleanse the body

These points will help this natural process of elimination of toxins to create balance and harmony within the body.

DU 20, Bai Hui (百会)

LI 11, Qu Qi (曲池)

EM 30, BaXie (八邪)

EM 45, BaFeng (八风)

RN 8, Shen Que (神阙) (breathing practice)

SP 6, San Yin Jiao (三阴交)

LR 3, Tai Chong (太冲)

KI 27, Shu Fu (俞府)

Massage at least once a month. After massage, drink plenty of water and you should be well-rested.

Facial Acupoints - For Beautiful skin

DU 20, Bai Hui (百会)

RN 23, Lian Quan (廉泉)

EX 2, Yin Tang (印堂)

DU 26, Ren Zhong (人中)

ST 2, Si Bai (四白)

ST 4, Di Cang (地仓)

BL 1, Jing Ming (睛明)

EX 2, Yin Tang (印堂)

EX 3, Tai Yang (太阳)

RN 24, Cheng Jiang (承浆)

SI 19, Ting Gong (听宫)

Clean your face well before massaging. Cream should be used. Make the message very gentle and never move from up to down, always massage upwards. The best time for this massage is before going to sleep at night.

Acupoints to strengthen the immune system

These points specifically target the immune system and will assist the body to resist viruses, such as colds, and flu, as well as more serious diseases.

RN 8, Shen Que (神阙)

SP 6, San Yin Jiao (三阴交)

LI 11, Qu Qi (曲池)

SI 6, Yang lao (养老)

KI 1, Yong Quan (涌泉)

KI 27, Shu Fu (俞府)

ST 36, Zu San Li (足三里)

SP 8, Di Ji (地机)

DU 4, Ming Men (命门)

Alleviating damage caused by sadness

Some people carry past sadness through their lives. These points will help to clear the sadness and boost happiness and positive energy. If you have temporary sadness, you can also clear it using your hand moving clockwise over the points and the area around the points.

RN 17, Dan Zhong (膻中)

EX 3, Tai Yang (太阳)

PC 6, Nei Guan (内关)

HT 7, Shen Men (神门)

LU 11, Shao Shang (少商)

LI 11, Qu Qi (曲池)

Acupoints to calm down and reduce anger

LR 3, Tai Chong (太冲)

EX 3, Tai Yang (太阳)

DU 20, Bai Hui (百会)

LI 11, Qu Qi (曲池)

PC 6, Nei Guan (内关)

HT 7, Shen Men (神门)

LI 4, He Gu (合谷)

Acupoints to reduce anxiety before an exam or interview

The first thing we need to do before the exam and interview is to be calm by breathing deeply and using these points. This will reduce stress to a minimum. This way you can avoid forgetfulness and ensure that the concentration works at the best level. To achieve this, you should start working one or two weeks before the exam.

DU 20, Bai Hui (百会)

PC 6, Nei Guan (内关)

HT 7, LI 4, He Gu (合谷)

EX 2, Yin Tang (印堂)

EX 3, Tai Yang (太阳)

Start a week or two before the exam or interview. Lie down, breathe deeply, massage the acupuncture points for 15-20 minutes with light music

Acupoints for Healthy and Beautiful Breasts

These acupoints protect the health of the breast by increasing the energy by keeping the blood circulation in the region in balance.

SP 21, Da Bao (大包)

SP 10, Xue Hai (血海)

ST 36, Zu San Li (足三里)

SP 6, San Yin Jiao (三阴交)

LR 3, Tai Chong (太冲)

RN 17, Dan Zhong (膻中)

Acupoints for Motion Sickness

These points are important to prevent and treat motion sickness in cars, boats, buses and planes.

PC 6, Nei Guan (内关)

LI 4, He Gu (合谷)

DU 26, Ren Zhong (人中)

DU 20, Bai Hui (百会)

Method of Application Before the trip, for protection, apply massage to each point 12-18 times in the form of light pressure for 3 consecutive days and a deep breath workout is performed for 10 minutes each day. During the trip, massage is applied by pressing or tapping.

Qi Gong

How Qi Gong and Qi Gong Energy Works

Qi Gong and Qi Gong Energy Mechanism are the types of exercises done to protect our body's health. The aim is to regulate the breath, body movement and consciousness. This long-term workout can have a big impact on human health if practised daily. It can also have a positive impact on mental and physical health.

Scientific research into Qi Gong is currently being undertaken. Over the years, scientists from both East and West have conducted scientific research into the energy production mechanisms in our bodies. Getting into deeper research of the human energy mechanisms have shown surprising results. In classic Qi Gong, 'Qi' means 'energy' and 'Gong' means 'ability' or 'earned'. Qi Gong research investigates the energy mechanism and how the energy earned is expanded or increased.

The Grey Condition

The Grey Condition is not part of Chinese Medicine however, as we discuss vital organs, I wish to cover it.

Good health is the cornerstone of all good life. It is a gift and a right for everybody. As technology and our lifestyle changes, the way humans define health is also changing.

Previously, health was known as 'no illness'. Now the definition is 'total physical, mental and social well-being'. In fact, health and wellbeing is a balanced state of movement and living.

The 10 health measure standards as follows:

1. Filled with energy, can carry out daily living and work without strain
2. Has a positive attitude and manners; is active; takes on duties without complaint
3. Quality sleeping
4. Has resistance against colds and flu
5. Has appropriate weight and has good posture
6. Has good eyesight and fast response and reflexes
7. Healthy, clean, painless teeth with normal non-bleeding gums
8. Has shiny, healthy hair
9. Has strong bones, filled muscles, and healthy skin elasticity

10. Can adjust to the environment; can face and tackle difficulties and can walk strong.

If we think about these, how many of us can say we are healthy? We can look and feel OK while still having sub-clinical (unobservable) health conditions. This is sometimes referred to as The Grey Condition.

Some causes include

1. The negative impact of the environment and living conditions
2. Disorderly living
3. Bad habits
4. Not practicing enough sport or doing enough exercise
5. Working under pressure and against the biological clock
6. Poor nutrition, noise, air pollution
7. Inappropriate use of medication
8. Stress
9. Emotions

They are associated with an imbalance of Yin and Yang. Needless to say, the grey condition will progress from sub-clinical to clinical if not addressed. Thus, the reason for this book.

My Affirmations

I would like to share with you the way I believe the relationship between health and success can support us.

By saying affirmations out loud every day, I improve my own health.

You can try it at home as well.

1. Because I am healthy, I am beautiful.
2. Because I am beautiful, I am confident.
3. Because I am confident, I am sincere.
4. Because I am sincere, I have good friends.
5. Because I have good friends, I am strong and able.
6. Because I am strong and able, I am successful.
7. Because I am successful, I can do more good things for humanity and this world!

My mother's advice for a healthy and happy life

1. Keep your waist and feet warm, but your head cool
2. Listen to the elders and children
3. Don't drink your tea too hot
4. Don't eat too much
5. Go to bed early and get up early
6. Be friendly, always be smiling for others.
7. Always say thank you to others
8. Don't stay in the wind with wet hair
9. Don't go out without breakfast
10. Claim and know your values
11. Don't forget to say hello to everyone
12. Share your joy with your friends
13. Always sit down to drink your water and juice
14. Don't be lazy, do something
15. When you get upset, meet your friend and share with them
16. After dinner, walk 100 steps
17. Always eat fondly
18. Have garlic on your journey, you won't be sick
19. Don't complain. Think about solutions and pray

16 Principles of Abundant Energy, Health and Wellbeing

1. Nature will cure, medicine is the servant of nature.
2. The human body is an organism and able to mend itself
3. Energy increases if used correctly.
4. Look for the cure in your heart
5. Pay attention to your body and soul to move together.
6. The best cure is love.
7. The answer to a smiling face is a smiling face.
8. If you want the world to smile at you, you need to see its beauty.
9. Use your precious breath correctly, it will always make you energetic and healthy.
10. Our bodies are perfect. Listen to your body. It will always tell you what to do.
11. Laughter is a marvellous medicine; it keeps us young and healthy.
12. Don't neglect to listen to music and feed your soul.
13. At least once a week, spare some time for yourself. Do something you like.
14. Recognise your own value – put the value first.
15. You matter.
16. Always be learning something new, doing something different.

AFTERWORD

In my 38 years of professional life, I have seen that people do not want to suffer while being treated. They do not want side effects and they want to regain their health easily.

If we learn the healing power of the acupoints - the prescription in our pocket - our health will benefit on a daily basis.

CASE STUDIES AND TESTIMONIALS

Case Studies

Loss of Appetite

A 23-year-old girl, preparing for university. To become more energetic, she started taking a few kinds of vitamins. After a while, her appetite began to diminish, she felt tired and nauseated. When she went to the doctor, who told her liver function had deteriorated, and she had to go to hospital.

Her family was thinking she would not recover. When I examined her, she looked very weak. I treated her with acupoint massage and applied Energy healing for her. One day after in the treatment she was asking for food.

The healing method of Chinese medicine is in principle the balancing of spleen and stomach energy. In this way, it supports the digestive system, which then works in a balanced way.

Aphonia

I once had the opportunity to treat Bjork, the world-famous singer. She was giving a concert in Istanbul in august 2008 a few years ago. A few days before the concert she had been suffering from aphonia (She had lost her voice with laryngitis). She found my number from my organiser and I treated her at the hotel the day she arrived. She didn't sleep the whole night after the therapy. But she understood and trusted that this therapy would benefit her, and she told me she was not worried at all. On the day after the second treatment, just a day later, she had a very successful concert.

Substance Abuse

A 25-year-old man came to me and said in a timid manner that he wanted to quit the substance he had been using for 11 years. I had never had a patient like this before, yet we both had faith that we could achieve success. We set out with courage, love, respect, and trust. Our treatment continued with acupuncture, bioenergy, Qi Gong, and life coaching. The Ra Qi therapy.

The young man was changing, his eyes began to shine, his hair began to shine, his skin began to colour, his posture began to be erect. He stopped using drugs.

At the end of 6 months, the drugs were eradicated from that body and we had reached the final conclusion. Sixteen years have passed, now he is a very successful businessman, team leader, a wonderful father and a husband who knows his responsibility.

–o0o–

Testimonials

Dr Veli is one of the most intuitive and insightful practitioners I have encountered. Her clinical approach is disarming as she carries with her a child-like spirit, while at the same time delivers professional treatments with conviction and clarity. She does not fall into the trap of over-reaching as she is comfortable saying "I don't know", yet she has a talent for inspiring reassurance and comfort. In a world of increasing stress and tension, her treatment would provide an integral part of any person's self-care protocol.

Dr Arthur Stabolidis Clinical Psychologist, Melbourne

...

I saw Ravza on a TV show and I immediately thought of my 12-year-old daughter. She still had urinary incontinence while sleeping at night (wetting the bed). I immediately called the program. You showed us the energy healing method I could do from home on the screen. It was very easy to do. I only had to treat my daughter 7-8 days at home and got wonderful results. It was an incredible thing. We had visited a lot of hospitals and used a lot of drugs for years, there was no result until then. I helped my daughter heal by treating her myself at home!

This incident inspired my daughter to work as a nurse and she is now working at that same hospital helping solve other people's problems. I send you my endless thanks!

Nurcan, 35-year-old women, Istanbul

...

Having been bedridden for months with no energy, no appetite, and a host of other mysterious symptoms, I was completely debilitated by an undiagnosed chronic illness and utterly hopeless when I first met Dr. Ravza. After our first session, my entire body went freezing on a hot midsummer day, with the heater on in the room and a wool blanket over me. After that initial acupuncture and massage therapy, I was up, walking again with my energy noticeably better and my appetite back (I could walk around the house and then sit up straight for several hours, and downed a whole banana!). Throughout the subsequent treatments, I watched my body regain its ability to heal itself with the help of Dr. Ravza's touch and needles. Our journey was nothing short of miraculous and awe-inspiring: one day, Dr. Ravza's body would take on my problems as the growls from my stomach would cease only to resurface in her stomach. On another day, she would not be able to hold her tears back as she treated me. Yet on another, she could not stop yawning throughout the entire session... all this, as my physical and mental toxic overload was unloading through her body.

If it were not for Dr. Ravza I would not have been able to take my chronic condition under control and have the beautiful life I lead now. My family and I are forever indebted to Dr. Ravza for the unceasing support and love she has provided us with for the past 10 years, even when continents away, and am thankful for her existence and for being such a strong pillar in my life.

Belin, 38-year-old women, Istanbul

...

I was experiencing excruciating migraine headaches which resulted in me going to different doctors throughout my life. The last doctor advised a medication that I was on for a while and later found out that this medication had very bad side effects and so I stopped taking it. I went through severe depression (including unstoppable thoughts of committing suicide and generally discontent with my life and myself), sleepless nights, anxiety and unstoppable tremors in different parts of my body.

This went on for months until I met Ravza at a seminar I attended as I was looking for natural therapy solutions to recover from these horrible side effects. After a number of sessions with her, including coaching, Ra-Qi therapy, and energy healing, my body slowly but surely started taking notice of and responding positively to these treatments. After a period of time and after a number of treatments, I was slowly beginning to get back on my feet and paying closer attention to my daily needs, sleeping better, having less tremors and gaining some normality back into my life. I felt calm but energetic and slowly began to feel the need to look after myself and my well-being.

Without Ravza's treatments and the support that she has provided, I would not be where I am today. I can't speak highly enough of Ravza and how much her treatments have empowered me to take control of my life.

Sayra 61-year-old woman, Melbourne

...

I was constantly feeling lethargic, angry, stressed, confused and always forgetting to do things. My mother kept telling me about how my actions were affecting those around me and how I needed to find ways to get over these feelings. At the time, my mother was receiving treatment from Ravza and so she encouraged me to see her also.

So, I agreed to meet Ravza. First, we had a coaching session, followed by a session of looking at different chakras of the body and finding out which parts of my body required urgent treatment. My sessions involved, cupping, acupuncture, Ra-Qi therapy and energy healing. I will never forget the day when I woke up from a deep state of meditation where I inhaled air into my lungs with almost no control and exhaled with great force.

Something had left my body for good. I finally knew what it was like to breathe. I felt light. I felt calm. I felt focused. Furthermore, I was sleeping better and feeling less tired. This didn't happen overnight, but it did happen after a number of treatments. Each time, I was feeling a little better, more relaxed, less anxious, more in control of my feelings and the feelings of those around me. I am so grateful to Ravza for helping me tap into my inner soul and re-connecting me with life in general.

Arya, 36-year-old woman, Melbourne

GLOSSARY

Abdomen	The part of the body internally between the diaphragm and the anus
Acupoints	Locations on the body susceptible to manipulation by needles or massage to elicit a healing response to various symptoms
Acupuncture	Stimulation of certain points on the skin by using needles to elicit a healing response to various symptoms
Anemia	Reduced capacity of the blood to transport oxygen
Anorexia	Loss of appetite
Anterior	Towards the front
Apoplexy	Bleeding within internal organs. An old term for a stroke.
Autonomic nervous System	The network of nerves that regulates unconscious functions such as breathing, heart beat and digestion.
Ayurveda	A form of Tibetan healing
Canthus	The inner or outer corner of the eye
Cardiac	Pertaining to the heart
Cun (pronounced 'choon')	A measure used for determining the location of acupuncture points. It varies from person to person, but is about 2.5 cm in an adult
Deficiency	In Chinese Medical terms deficiency implies reduced function of and organ, system, blood, or Qi.
Diaphragm	The band of muscle separating the abdomen from the thorax. The diaphragm controls breathing
Distal	Further away from the centre

Dysmenorrhea	Painful menstruation
Edema	Swelling brought about by accumulation of fluid
Enuresis	Involuntary urination
Erysipelas	A skin infection
Fibula	The narrow bone in the lower leg next to the tibia.
Five Element Theory	A theory in Chinese Medicine that suggests there are 5 interacting aspects of entities such as body organs, colours, and emotions.
Fu organs	The six hollow organs – stomach, large intestine, small intestine, bladder, and San Jiao (Triple Burner)
Hypertension	High blood pressure
Hypotension	Low blood pressure
Insomnia	Inability to sleep
Lateral	On the side
Libido	Desire to have sex, sex drive
Lymphatic system	A system of vessels within the body that clears toxins and cellular debris.
Malleolus	The inner or outer protrusive bone of the ankle
Medial	Towards the centre
Meridian	A purported channel within the body that carries Qi and links the organs.
Metacarpal	Any one of the bones of the hand
Metacarpophalangeal joint	The knuckle at the base of the finger
Metatarsal	Any one of the bones in the foot
Metatarsophalangeal joint	The joint at the base of the toe
Moxa	A herb (mugwort) that practitioners use to exerts a therapeutic effect by burning

Moxibustion	The method of burning a dried herb called Moxa used in conjunction with needles or on its own at various acupoints Stimulation of certain points on the skin by using needles to elicit a healing response to various symptoms
Neurological	Pertaining to the nerves
Pericardium	A protective tissue surrounding the heart
Posterior	Towards the back
Proximal	Closer to the centre
Qi	According to Chinese Medicine, Qi is energy that drives motion of the body and function of the organs.
Ra Qi	A treatment modality incorporating aspects of acupuncture, massage and reiki, created by Dr Ravza Veli.
Radius	The rotating bone of the forearm
San Jiao	A name given to the functions the three sections of the abdomen - upper, middle, and lower.
Symptom	A physiological or behavioural indication of an ailment or disease
Temporal	In the area of the temples
Thenar eminence	The ball of the thumb
Thorax	The chest cavity
Tibia	What we call the shin bone
Tinnitus	Ringing in the ears
Trigeminal neuralgia	Facial pain cause by disturbance of the trigeminal nerve.
Tui Na	A massage technique of Chinese Medicine
Ulna	The fixed bone of the forearm
Umbilicus	The navel
Unilateral	On one side
Uticaria	A rash

Vertebra	A joint of the spine
Vertigo	Dizziness
Wei Qi	Protective Qi that repels invasive pathogens
Yin and Yang	A traditional Chinese philosophy wherein opposites are considered to be opposite and complementary parts of a quality or entity. e.g. male/female, light/dark, heat/cold.
Ying Qi	The Qi derived from food and drink
Yuan Qi	The vital energy with which we are born
Zang organs	The five solid organs - lungs, liver, heart, spleen, and kidneys
Zong Qi	Qi provided by nature from breathing air

ABOUT THE AUTHOR

Dr. Ravza Yausheva Veli was born in Urumchi, China. Her early childhood years were spent in Beijing where her family lived and worked. In 1976, she gained entry to the Xin Jiang Medical University where she studied medicine.

After graduating she became a Radiology specialist at Xin Jiang Autonomous Regional Hospital, while continuing her research work on Traditional Chinese Medicine (TCM).

In 1991, she presented as a guest lecturer at the Aegean University in Turkey, and also held seminars on acupuncture and Chinese Massage (Tui Na) at the Ege University, where she studied Turkish language for six months.

In 1997 Dr Veli opened her own clinic where she worked in acupuncture, energy healing, points massage and aromatherapy for many years.

Here she honed her healing skills and became a renowned speaker and presentered on the subject on television for various health program. Among the thousands of people, she has treated over many years, she has also worked with Bjork, Massive Attack, Rhianna's band and the cast of Mama Mia as they travelled and performed in Istanbul, Turkey.

Dr. Veli has presented at various international and professional conferences, including the Acupuncture Congress in China, USA and Turkey, and the International Congress for dermatologists for Turkish speakers and the Ethno-music Therapist Congress in Istanbul over many years.

Dr. Veli also trained as an aesthetician and beauty therapist in Turkey. Since 2007, she has given seminars to communities in Austria, Australia, USA and Kazan, Russia. She currently speaks at seminars and runs courses about 'Health through the Acupoints' and 'The miracle points in our bodies'.

As owner and founder of the Dr. Ravza Wellbeing Centre in Melbourne, her mission is to help people to learn to strengthen their immune system in order to prevent disease. She gives regular seminars on health and healing as well as Self -Help in English, Turkish, Tatar and Uyghur languages.

She is married and has one son and a granddaughter.

Printed in the United States
By Bookmasters